Immune Depression and Cancer

[Irwin Strasburger Memorial Seminar
on Immunology, 2d, Cornell University Medical College, 1975.

IMMUNE DEPRESSION AND CANCER

PROCEEDINGS OF THE SECOND IRWIN STRASBURGER MEMORIAL SEMINAR ON IMMUNOLOGY

EDITED BY

Gregory W. Siskind, M.D.
Charles L. Christian, M.D.
Stephen D. Litwin, M.D.

SPONSORED BY

The Department of Medicine

CORNELL UNIVERSITY MEDICAL COLLEGE
THE NEW YORK HOSPITAL
NEW YORK, NEW YORK 10021

RC262
A1
I 76
1975

GRUNE & STRATTON
A Subsidiary of Harcourt Brace Jovanovich, Publishers
New York   San Francisco   London

311218

Library of Congress Cataloging in Publication Data

Irwin Strasburger Memorial Seminar on Immunology, 2d,
    Cornell University Medical College, 1975.
    Immune depression and cancer.

    1. Cancer—Immunological aspects—Congresses.
2. Immunosuppressive agents—Congresses.
I. Siskind, Gregory W.   II. Christian, Charles L.,
1926-   III. Litwin, Stephen D.   IV. Cornell
University. Dept. of Medicine.   V. Title.
[DNLM: 1.   Neoplasms—Immunology—Congresses.
 2.   Immunosuppression—Congresses.   W3 IR72 1974i /
QZ200 I72 1973i]
RC262.I76   1975   616.9′94′079   75-22110

© *1975 by Grune & Stratton, Inc.*
All rights reserved. No part of this publication
may be reproduced or transmitted in any form or
by any means, electronic or mechanical, including
photocopy, recording, or any information storage
and retrieval system, without permission in
writing from the publisher.

Grune & Stratton, Inc.
111 Fifth Avenue
New York, New York 10003

Library of Congress Catalog Number 75-22110
International Standard Book Number 0-8089-0910-X
Printed in the United States of America

CONTENTS

ACKNOWLEDGMENTS

The symposium was made possible by a gift from The Irwin Strasburger Memorial Medical Foundation.

This photo-ready book was designed and typed by Miss Antoinette Sapienza.

The discussions following the presentations and the discussion by Dr. Hans Wigzell were transcribed and edited from tape recordings made during the symposium.

PREFACE

These symposia arose through a suggestion of Dr. J. Russell Twiss, Medical Director of The Irwin Strasburger Memorial Medical Foundation and long time staff member of The New York Hospital. The symposia became a reality through the generous financial support of the Irwin Strasburger Memorial Medical Foundation. The purpose of the symposia is to bring together each year outstanding medical scientists to discuss current aspects of problems related to both immunology and cancer. The selection of the topic for this year, *Immune Depression and Cancer,* was initiated by the increasing level of serious investigation concerned with manipulation of the immune response and its relationship to malignancies and medical practice. The selection of speakers represents an attempt to touch on critical issues and highlights of the field rather than to survey all present knowledge.

A final note concerns the late Irwin Strasburger, a philanthropist, who was concerned about the support of medical research especially in the area of neoplastic disease. The Irwin Strasburger Memorial Medical Foundation came into existence as a result of efforts by Dr. J. Russell Twiss with the support of Mr. Strasburger's wife, family, and friends. The Foundation was designed to serve as a memorial to Mr. Strasburger's memory by supporting work and education in the area of his interests.

The first Irwin Strasburger Memorial Seminar was held at Cornell University Medical College on October 29, 1973 and dealt with Basic Immunology and Cancer.

CONTRIBUTORS

Symposium on Immune Depression and Cancer held at Cornell University Medical College, New York City, on February 3, 1975.

ALAN C. AISENBERG
John Collins Warren Laboratories of the Huntington
Memorial Hospital of Harvard University at
The Massachusetts General Hospital,
Boston, Massachusetts.

WILLIAM Q. ASCARI
Somerset Hospital, Somerville, New Jersey and
Ortho Diagnostic Research Foundation,
Raritan, New Jersey.

SIDNEY R. COOPERBAND
Boston University School of Medicine,
Boston, Massachusetts.

RICHARD K. GERSHON
Yale University School of Medicine,
New Haven, Connecticut.

DAVID H. KATZ
Department of Pathology, Harvard Medical School,
Boston, Massachusetts.

GREGORY W. SISKIND
Division of Allergy and Immunology, Department of
Medicine, Cornell University Medical College,
New York, New York.

ALFRED D. STEINBERG
National Institutes of Health, Bethesda, Maryland.

THOMAS A. WALDMANN
Metabolism Branch, National Cancer Institute,
National Institutes of Health, Bethesda, Maryland.

DISCUSSANT

DR. HANS WIGZELL
The Wallenberg Laboratory, University of Uppsala
Uppsala, Sweden

SUPPRESSOR T CELLS: CLASSES OF ACTIVITY

Richard K. Gershon

Yale University School of Medicine
New Haven, Connecticut

INTRODUCTION

Although the early studies of interactions between subpopulations of lymphocytes emphasized the positive side of
the interaction effects, a body of evidence has been
accumulating over the past few years which indicates that
negative interaction effects may be of equal importance in
immunoregulation (1-5). In particular T cells have been
shown to suppress the immune response in a number of diverse
situations. In those situations where T cells act to suppress
the immune response they are called "suppressor T cells". It
is important to emphasize that this is an operational term
only; it has not been shown that suppressor T cells are a
distinct class or sub-line of cells. It seems more likely
(and economical) to think of T cells as regulatory cells which
can either amplify or suppress the immune response. Which
course they choose to take depends on a number of factors,
but is probably a result of signal discrimination at the cell
level rather than a conflict between two different cells (1).
However, once the signal discrimination has occurred and a
T cell has differentiated towards suppression this differentiated cell appears to become committed and can be separated
from other T cells.

It would be useful at this juncture of the evolution of
our understanding of immunoregulation by T cells to review
and classify the available body of evidence on suppressor
T cells. What follows is an attempt to do this.

1

DISCUSSION

I. IMMUNOLOGICAL TOLERANCE

   A. *Direct: Suppression by T Cells.*

        Certain states of acquired immunologic tolerance
have been shown to be "infectious" in that cells from
putatively tolerant animals can cause normal cells to become
specifically unresponsive (5-16). This specific suppressor
phenomenon is totally thymic dependent in both its inductive
and effector phases. Specific suppressor T-cell effects
have been demonstrated with cells from non-tolerant animals
as well (17-27). They are operative in high and low zone
tolerance, affect antibody and cell-mediated responses, can
be activated by soluble or particulate antigens, and can
exhibit hapten or carrier specificity. Some investigators
have been unable to show "infectious" suppression by mixing
tolerant and normal cells, which may suggest that suppressor
T cells are not active in all types of tolerance (28,29).
However, in one case where cells from tolerant animals
failed to produce "infectious suppression" in mixture type
experiments, it was also impossible to break tolerance by
adoptive transfer of normal cells into the tolerant animals
(28). Although the reasons for this failure were not
determined, it is possible that suppressor cells were
involved. For reasons not entirely clear it is always much
easier to demonstrate suppression by transferring cells into
a suppressive environment than by transferring the suppressor
cells into a new or neutral environment (1,31,31).

   B. *Indirect: T-Cell Dependence of Specific B-Cell
Unresponsiveness.*

        Presentation of antigen to B cells which are
incapable of responding by antibody production, due to the
removal of T cells, fails to induce a state of tolerance
(27,32-36). In several instances the same antigen presentation produced a state of specific B-cell unresponsiveness
if T cells were present during the induction period (27,32,
35,36). Although these results are compatible with the
notion that B-cell tolerance depends on suppressor T-cell
activity, there are a number of discordant results and
complicating factors which may make such an interpretation

hazardous. I will discuss this point in greater detail below.

II. ANTIGENIC COMPETITION

Antigenic competition, the phenomenon by which inoculation of one antigen non-specifically interferes with the subsequently induced immune response to a second antigen, has been shown to be thymus dependent (37-38). Thus, a modest reduction of an animal's T-cell complement, which does not greatly affect its antibody response, can abrogate antigenic competition. This phenomenon, like immunological tolerance, was shown to be an active immunosuppressive event. Normal cells given to an animal in whom antigenic competition is occurring become inactivated, and subject to the milieu effect (31,37-39). Antibody production is not required for this effect, since passively administered antibody to the first (competing) antigen may inhibit antibody production against this antigen, while allowing the competitive event to occur undampened (40). It is important to emphasize that this non-specific thymus-dependent form of suppression has not been shown to be directly mediated by a T-cell produced factor: the indirect participation of thymus dependent macrophages has been implicated in some cases (41). Further, it has not been conclusively demonstrated that the T cell (or the T-dependent macrophage) makes a factor which is directly suppressive. Feldmann has suggested the possibility of an indirect suppression produced by the occupancy (saturation) of essential cooperating sites on macrophages by T-cell helper factors, induced by and specific for the first antigen (42).

More recently, several new types of non-specific T-cell dependent suppression have been described which are probably related to antigenic competition and which suggest that activated T cells do release factors which directly suppress other immunologically competent cells.

A. *Mitogen Activated T-Cells.*

Subpopulations of Con A activated T cells release a highly immunosuppressive factor (43-46). Studies of its mode of action make it seem highly unlikely that it works by

blocking macrophages; there is a considerable latent period
after it is added to culture before its suppressive effect
is seen (46). Similar latencies have been noted in other
studies on suppressor T cells (6,47-48). This delay in
action of suppressor T-cell factors could explain why
transient immune responses are often seen during tolerance
induction.

B. *Cultured T Cells.*

Educated thymic T cells cultured for a six to eight
hour period with the specific antigen used for education
acquire the ability to suppress the specific response of
normal cells, as well as non-specific responses, if specific
antigen is present (49). The "specific" effect of a non-
specific suppressor cannot be explained by a macrophage
saturation mechanism. Interestingly, during the six to
eight hour cultivation period the educated T cells release
a specific cooperating factor into the supernatant. The
relationship of the loss of this factor from the cultured
cells to the appearance of the suppressors is unclear but
appears to be a fruitful area for investigation. It has
previously been suggested that suppressor activity can be
masked by "contrasuppressor" activity (50). This may be a
case where suppressor activity is unmasked by loss of contra-
suppression.

C. *Spleen Seeking T Cells.*

Splenic and thymic T cells which localize in the
spleen can exert a pronounced suppressive effect on ongoing
immune responses in the lymph nodes (2,47,51). T cells
harvested from lymph nodes do not appear to have similar
suppressive effects when they localize in the spleen,
suggesting that this effect may be mediated by a distinct
T-cell subpopulation rather than being a phenomenon induced
by the microenvironment (2,51). Another argument against
microenvironmental induction is the ability of antigen
activated splenic T cells to suppress *in vitro* responses,
while lymph node T cells from the same animal help the
response (52,54). This *in vitro* effect of splenic T cells
appears to have the same specificity and induction require-
ments as the educated cultured T cells described above.

The observation that spleen seeking T cells exert immunosuppressive effects may be particularly revelent to tumor immunology. The immunosuppressive role of the spleen in the response to tumors has been well established, although the mechanism by which it exerts its immunosuppressive influence is unknown (reviewed in 55). Suppressor T cells have been shown to modulate the immune response to tumors (56-59). That they may be the important regulatory cells in the spleens of tumor bearing mice is suggested by the bidirectional nature of the splenic regulation; that is the effect of splenectomy on the immune response to a tumor graft depends to some extent on the size of the graft (60). {See section VII below on feedback regulation.} Thus, the spleen has been shown to suppress the response to large tumor grafts and increase the response to smaller grafts.

III. AUTOIMMUNITY

Monier (61) and Allison (62,63) have reviewed evidence suggesting that T cells may have a prophylactic role in prevention of autoimmune disease. In particular, T-cell depletion may hasten and increase the appearance of auto-antibodies and autoimmune diseases in some strains of mice, rats and chickens. Inoculations of normal T cells may delay or prevent their occurrence. In addition, spleen cells from young but not older NZB mice are highly prone to develop autoimmune disease. Their thymic T cells have also been noted to be deficient in immunoregulatory functions (65). Lastly, it has recently been recognized that thymusless nude mice are particularly prone to develop autoantibodies (66-68).

IV. CLASS SPECIFIC T-CELL SUPPRESSION

Tada and his associates (69-72) have reported that the homocytotrophic dinitrophenyl (DNP) antibody response of rats immunized with DNP-Ascaris could be increased by a number of maneuvers which deplete T-cells. This enhanced response could be rapidly abrogated by the inoculation of thymocytes from syngeneic rats hyperimmunized to either Ascaris or DNP-Ascaris, whereas cells from rats hyperimmunized to DNP-bovine serum albumin (BSA) were without effect. These experiments virtually rule out antibody as a causative agent as the carrier (Ascaris) immune cells were suppressive while

anticarrier antibody was not. In addition, the same carrier
specificity for T-cell suppression was shown as had previously been shown for T-cell help. Kishimoto and Ishizaka
(73) have shown similar class specific antibody suppression
in vitro.

V.   AUGMENTATION OF THYMUS INDEPENDENT IMMUNE RESPONSES

There are some antigens which fail to activate any
demonstrable helper T-cell activity in normal animals (1,74).
The immune response to these antigens can be augmented by a
variety of means which reduce the T-cell complement (75-76).
The augmented response may be diminished by restoration of
thymocytes (76). This augmentation appears to be thymus
dependent in that excessive T-cell reduction prevents the
augmentation (17). Thus, it seems that the reason this class
of antigens seems to exhibit thymus independence in their
immune response is because they activate suppressor T cells
preferentially, and that the target of the T-cell suppression
is other T cells and not B cells. A similar situation seems
to obtain in other special situations, which are regulated by
Ir genes (see next section).

VI.   CONTROL OF GENETICALLY DETERMINED IMMUNOLOGICAL UNRESPONSIVENESS

A gene or genes closely linked to those which determine
histocompatibility has (have) been shown in a number of
species to determine the capacity to make an immune response
to certain well-defined antigens (77). In at least one such
case, the basis for this form of specific immunological unresponsiveness has been shown to be that the T cells of non-
responder animals have an inordinate propensity to become
tolerant to the antigen in question (78). This form of
tolerance in addition to the others detailed above has been
shown to be governed by suppressor T cells (79), and to
have T cells as targets (J. Ordal, S. Smith, F.C. Grumet
and R.K. Gershon, in preparation).

VII. FEEDBACK REGULATION

A. *From T Cells.*

T cells respond to antigen with a circumscribed
period of DNA synthesis (80,81). The amount of DNA synthesized, as well as the duration of the period of DNA synthesis, is determined in part by regulatory interactions
between the responding cells (47,81-84). Non-antigen
responsive T cells may also regulate the response in a
fashion which suggests that they recognize signals from the
responding cells; that is, the same population of non-
antigen responsive regulatory cells can act to augment low
responses and suppress higher responses (2,47,82-84).

B. *From B Cells.*

B cell products, in particular antibody, can both
inhibit or augment immune responses (85). At least some of
these regulatory functions are mediated indirectly by T cells
(86), which seem to be able to sense the level of B-cell
activity and regulate the subsequent antibody response in a
fashion quite similar to the way they regulate the response
of other T cells (87).

VIII. REGULATION OF NON-ANTIGEN INDUCED EVENTS

A. *Allotype Suppression.*

Allotype suppression, in which exposure of the
neonate to antibody against allotypic determinants on its
own immunoglobulins suppresses production of those immunoglobulins, has been found to exhibit T-cell dependence in
some circumstances (3).

B. *Immunoglobulin Production.*

Peripheral blood B cells from humans with common
variable hypogammaglobulinemia fail to make significant
amounts of any immunoglobulin when cultured with pokeweed
mitogen, while cells from normal controls do (4). Mixtures
of cells from different normal controls respond to pokeweed
quite normally, while mixtures of normal and hypogammaglobulinemic cells fail to respond. The suppressor cell in the

peripheral blood of the hypogammaglobulinemic patients was shown to have T-cell characteristics.

It has also been shown that bone marrow cells from chickens rendered agammaglobulinemic by bursectomy and irradiation contain similar suppressor cells although their T-cell origin is less well established in this case (88). It is of note, however, that the richest source of allotype suppressor T cells is mouse bone marrow (89). This may be related to the fact that the bone marrow is where the action is or, more interestingly, it may be that there is a sub-population of bone marrow seeking T cells with a special function of regulating B-cell differentiation.

CONCLUSIONS

The numerous and diverse situations in which suppressor T-cell activity has been reported, as noted in this brief review, suggest that these cells play a very important role in immunoregulation. Determining precisely how, why, when and where they work will be formidable tasks and should keep cellular immunologists quite busy during the next decade.

ACKNOWLEDGEMENTS

This research has been funded by USPHS grants CA-08593 from the NCI and AI-10497 from the NIAID.

I am also pleased to acknowledge the contributions of my many colleagues who helped in the work reported, who are annotated in the references.

REFERENCES

1. Gershon, R.K., Contemp. Topics Immunobiol., *3*: 1, 1974.

2. Gershon, R.K., in *The Immune System: Genes, Receptors, Signals*, Edited by E. Sercarz, A. Williamson and C.F. Fox, p. 471, Academic Press, New York, 1974.

3. Herzenberg, L.A. and Herzenberg, L.A., Contemp. Topics Immunobiol., *3*: 41, 1974.

4. Waldmann, T.A., Durm, M., Broder, S., Blackman, M., Blaese, R.M. and Strober, W., Lancet, *2*: 609, 1974.

5. Gershon, R.K. and Kondo, K., Immunology, *21*: 903, 1971.

6. McCullagh, P.J., J. Exp. Med., *132*: 916, 1970.

7. Zembala, M. and Asherson, G.L., Nature, *244*: 227, 1973.

8. Weber, G. and Kolsch, E., Eur. J. Immunol., *3*: 767, 1973

9. Ada, G.L. and Cooper, M.G., in *Immunological Tolerance: Mechanisms and Potential Therapeutic Applications*, Edited by D.H. Katz and B. Benacerraf, p. 87, Academic Press, New York, 1974.

10. Baker, P., Stashak, P.W., Amsbaugh, D.F. and Prescott,B., J. Immunol., *112*: 2020, 1974.

11. Basten, A., Miller, J.F.A.P., Sprent, J. and Cheers, C., J. Exp. Med., *140*: 199, 1974.

12. Claman, H.N., Phanuphak, T. and Morrhead, J.W., in *Immunological Tolerance: Mechanisms and Potential Therapeutic Applications*, Edited by D.H. Katz and B. Benacerraf, p. 123, Academic Press, New York, 1974.

13. Huchet, R. and Feldmann, M., Eur. J. Immunol., *4*: 768, 1974.

14. Waksman, B.H., in *Immunological Tolerance: Mechanisms and Potential Therapeutic Applications,* Edited by D.H. Katz and B. Benacerraf, p. 431, Academic Press, New York, 1974.

15. Rouse, B.T. and Warner, N.L., J. Immunol., *113*: 904, 1974.

16. Zan-Bar, I., Nachtigal, D. and Feldmann, M., Cell. Immunol., *10*: 19, 1974 (and personal communication).

17. Baker, P.J., Burns, W.H., Prescott, B., Stashak, P.W. and Amsbaugh, D.F., in *Immunological Tolerance: Mechanisms and Potential Therapeutic Applications,* Edited by D.H. Katz and B. Benacerraf, p. 493, Academic Press, New York, 1974.

18. Droege, W., Current Titles in Immunology, Transplantation and Allergy, *1*: 95 and 131, 1973.

19. Droege, W., in *The Immune System: Genes, Receptors, Signals,* Edited by E. Sercarz, A. Williamson and C.F. Fox, p. 431, Academic Press, New York, 1974.

20. Feldmann, M., Nature (New Biol.), *242*: 84, 1973.

21. Feldmann, M., Eur. J. Immunol., *4:* 660, 1974.

22. Feldmann, M., Eur. J. Immunol., *4*: 667, 1974.

23. Ha, T.Y. and Waksman, B.H., J. Immunol., *110*: 1290, 1973

24. Okumura, K. and Tada, T., Nature (New Biol.), *245*: 180, 1973.

25. Tada, T., in *Immunological Tolerance: Mechanisms and Potential Therapeutic Applications,* Edited by D.H. Katz and B. Benacerraf, p. 471, Academic Press, New York, 1974.

26. Elson, C.J. and Taylor, R.B., Eur. J. Immunol., *4*: 682, 1974.

27. Waldmann, H. and Munro, A.J., Eur. J. Immunol., *4*: 410, 1974.

28. Chiller, J.M. and Weigle, W.O., J. Immunol., *110*: 1051, 1973.

29. Scott, D.W., in *Immunological Tolerance: Mechanisms and Potential Therapeutic Applications,* Edited by D.H. Katz and B. Benacerraf, p. 503, Academic Press, New York, 1974.

30. Dwyer, J.M. and Kantor, F.S., J. Exp. Med., *137*: 32, 1973.

31. Waterston,R.H., Science, *170*: 1108, 1970.

32. Gershon, R.K. and Kondo, K., Immunology, *18*: 723, 1970.

33. Roelants, G.E. and Askonas, B.A., Nature (New Biol.), *239*: 63, 1973.

34. Davie, J.M. and Paul, W.E., J. Immunol., *113*: 1439, 1974.

35. Phillips-Quagliata, J.M., Bensinger, D.O. and Quagliata, F., J. Immunol., *111*: 1712, 1973.

36. Taylor, R.B. and Elson, C.J., in *Immunological Tolerance: Mechanisms and Potential Therapeutic Applications,* Edited by D.H. Katz and B. Benacerraf, p. 203, Academic Press, New York, 1974.

37. Gershon, R.K. and Kondo, K., J. Immunol., *106*: 1524, 1971.

38. Monier, J.-C., *Controle par le Thymus et les Cellules T., des Phenomenes D'Auto-Immunisation et de Competition Antigenique,* Ediprim, Lyon, 1972.

39. Menkes, J.S., Hencin, R.S. and Gershon, R.K., J. Immunol., *109*: 1052, 1972.

40. Gershon, R.K. and Kondo, K., J. Immunol., *106*: 1532, 1971.

41. Sjöberg, O., Clin. Exp. Immunol., *12*: 365, 1972.

42. Feldmann, M., J. Exp. Med., *136*: 737, 1972.

43. Dutton, R.W., J. Exp. Med., *136*: 1445, 1972.

44. Rich, R.R. and Pierce, C.W., J. Exp. Med., *137*: 649, 1973.

45. Dutton, R.W., J. Exp. Med., *138*: 1496, 1973.

46. Rich, R.R. and Pierce, C.W., J. Immunol., *112:* 1360, 1974.

47. Gershon, R.K., Lance, E.M. and Kondo, K., J. Immunol., *112*: 546, 1974.

48. Baker, P.J., Prescott, B., Stashak, P.W. and Amsbaugh, D.F., in *The Immune System: Genes, Receptors, Signals,* Edited by E. Sercarz, A. Williamson and C.F. Fox, p. 415, Academic Press, New York, 1974.

49. Taussig, M.J., Nature, *248*: 236, 1974.

50. Gershon, R.K., in *Immunological Tolerance: Mechanisms and Potential Therapeutic Applications,* Edited by D.H. Katz and B. Benacerraf, p. 441, Academic Press, New York, 1974.

51. Wu, C.-Y. and Lance, E.M., Cell. Immunol., *13*: 1, 1974.

52. Folch, H. and Waksman, B.H., J. Immunol., *113*: 127, 1974.

53. Folch, H. and Waksman, B.H., J. Immunol., *113*: 140, 1974.

54. Rich, S.S. and Rich, R.R., J. Exp. Med., *140*: 1588, 1974.

55. Gershon, R.K., Isr. J. Med. Sci., *10*: 1012, 1974.

56. Kirkwood, J.M. and Gershon, R.K., Prog. Exp. Tumor Res., *19*: 757, 1974.

57. Treves, A.J., Carnaud, C., Trainin, N., Feldmann, M. and Cohen, I.R., Eur. J. Immunol., *4*: 722, 1974.

58. Umiel, T. and Trainin, N., Transplantation, *18*: 244, 1974.

59. Schwartz, A. and Gershon, R.K., In Preparation.

60. Nordlund, J.J. and Gershon, R.K., J. Immunol., In Press.

61. Monier, J.-C., *Controle par le Thymus et les Cellules T., des Phenomenes d'Auto-Immunisation et de Competition Antigenique,* Ediprim, Lyon, 1972.

62. Allison, A.C., Contemp. Topics in Immunobiol., *3*: 227, 1974.

63. Allison, A.C., in *Immunological Tolerance: Mechanisms and Potential Therapeutic Applications,* Edited by D.H. Katz and B. Benacerraf, p. 25, Academic Press, New York, 1974.

64. Hardin, J.A., Chused, T.M. and Steinberg, A.D., J. Immunol., *111*: 650, 1973.

65. Dauphinee, M.J. and Talal, N., Proc. Nat. Acad. Sci. (U.S.), *70*: 3769, 1973.

66. Pantelouris, E.M., in *Proc. First Int. Workshop on Nude Mice,* Edited by J. Pygaard and C.O. Poolsen, p. 235, Fisher Verlag, Stuttgart, 1974.

67. Monier, J.-C., Sepetjian, M., Czyba, J.C., Ortonne, J.P. and Thivolet, J., in *Proc. First Int. Workshop on Nude Mice,* Edited by J. Pygaard and C.O. Poolsen, p. 243, Fisher Verlag, Stuttgart, 1974.

68. Morel,Maroger, L. and Salomon, J.-C., in *Proc. First Int. Workshop on Nude Mice,* Edited by J. Pygaard and C.O. Poolsen, p. 251, Fisher Verlag, Stuttgart, 1974.

69. Tada, T., Taniguchi, M. and Okumura, K., J. Immunol., *106*: 1012, 1971.

70. Taniguchi, T. and Tada, T., J. Immunol., *107*: 579, 1971.

71. Okumura, L. and Tada, T., J. Immunol., *106*: 1019, 1971.

72. Okumura, L. and Tada, T., J. Immunol., *107*: 1682, 1971.

73. Kishimoto, T. and Ishizaka, K., J. Immunol., *112*: 1685, 1974.

74. Kruger, J. and Gershon, R.K., J. Immunol., *108*: 581, 1972.

75. Kerbel, R.S. and Eidinger, D., Eur. J. Immunol., *2*: 114, 1972.

76. Baker, P.J., Stashak, P.W., Amsbaugh, D.F., Prescott, B. and Barth, R.J., Immunology, *105*: 1581, 1970.

77. Benacerraf, B. and McDevitt, H.O., Science, *175*: 273, 1972.

78. Gershon, R.K., Maurer, P.H. and Merryman, C.F., Proc. Nat. Acad. Sci. (U.S.), *70*: 250, 1973.

79. Benacerraf, B., Kapp, J.A. and Pierce, C.W., in *Immunological Tolerance: Mechanisms and Potential Therapeutic Applications,* Edited by D.H. Katz and B. Benacerraf, p. 507, Academic Press, New York, 1974.

80. Davies, A.J.S., Transpl. Rev., *1*: 43, 1969.

81. Gershon, R.K. and Liebhaber, S.A., J. Exp. Med., *136*: 112, 1972.

82. Gershon, R.K., Cohen, P., Hencin, R. and Liebhaber, S.A., J. Immunol., *108*: 586, 1972.

83. Gershon, R.K., Liebhaber, S.A. and Rye, S., Immunology, *26*: 909, 1974.

84. Gershon, R.K., in *Immunological Tolerance: Mechanisms and Potential Therapeutic Applications,* Edited by D.H. Katz and B. Benacerraf, p. 413, Academic Press, New York, 1974.

85. Uhr, J.W. and Möller, G., Adv. Immunol., *8*: 81, 1968.

86. Gershon, R.K., Mitchell, M.S. and Mokyr, M.B., Nature, *250*: 594, 1974.

87. Gershon, R.K., Orback-Arbouys, S. and Calkins, C., Proc. Second Int. Cong. Immunol., In Press.

88. Blaese, R.M., Weiden, P.L., Koski, I. and Dooley, N., J. Exp. Med., *140*: 1097, 1974.

89. Herzenberg, L.A. and Metzler, C.M., in, *Immunological Tolerance: Mechanisms and Potential Therapeutic Applications*, Edited by D.H. Katz and B. Benacerraf, p. 519, Academic Press, New York, 1974.

DISCUSSION FOLLOWING PRESENTATION

by DR. RICHARD K. GERSHON

G. SISKIND: On the basis of the differential localization
of suppressor T cells do you believe that there are two
different classes of T cells, one of which has suppressor
and one of which has helper activity or do you believe
that these functions are carried out by the same cell
under different physiologic conditions?

R. GERSHON: I do not think that there is any information
available that rules either hypothesis in or out. It is
quite clear that the suppressor T cell, when it is
suppressing, is doing something different from what is
done by a helper cell. The question is was it pre-
programed to do that before antigen exposure, or was it
able to read one or more signals and make a decision at
the time of antigen exposure. I think that there is no
information that can decide between these two possibilities at the moment. There are subpopulations of T cells
particularly immature T cells, which many workers have
found to more likely have suppressor than helper
activity. Whether these cells are the actual
suppressors, or whether they given signals to another
cell which does the actual suppressing cannot be decided
at this time. I should mention that neonatal animals
are just loaded with suppressor T cells. The reason
they make poor immune responses is because their T cells
suppress the response to any antigen you inject into
them. If you eliminate their T cells, their B cells
appear perfectly normal. This is reasonable since this
is the time when animals are developing immunological
tolerance against self antigens. These considerations
might suggest that there are really cells which are
programmed to be suppressors. However, I feel that
we should keep this question open at the present time.

I. SIEGEL: Are suppressor cells involved in self tolerance?

R. GERSHON: There are some peculiar antigens which can
    suppress B cells directly. However, most standard
    antigens do not seem to be able to directly suppress
    B cells. In the nude mouse, in contrast to other mice,
    you seem to he able to suppress B cells directly with
    antigen. There are several explanations for this. The
    concept which I favor is that very immature B cells can
    be paralyzed by the presence of large amounts of
    antigen. After they mature beyond a certain point, they
    can no longer be directly rendered tolerant. If this is
    true, there will certainly be elimination of immature
    B cells by exposure to self antigens. However, there
    appear to be large numbers of cells that can make
    products against self which are not eliminated. The
    activity of these cells seems to be controlled by
    suppressor T cells.

J. SCHRADER: Could the difference between the immune T-cell
    population and the normal T-cell population be a
    difference in number of cells?

R. GERSHON: The answer is no. We have gone throughout the
    dose response curve and the more normal T cells you add
    the more suppression you observe. It just plateaus out,
    it never turns into help. If you get enough immune
    T cells they will suppress so that there is an element
    of "superhelp" being suppressive. However, in the case
    where you are titrating out the B cells of immune or
    normal animals it is not a matter of dose. There is a
    qualitative difference in both the T cells and B cells.

QUESTION: You said that there was no such thing as a T-
    independent antigen. What do you mean by that statement?

R. GERSHON: What I mean is that there is no such thing as an
    antigen for which there is no T-cell recognition.
    There are antibody responses in which T cells do not
    participate, possibly as a result of suppressor
    mechanisms. As far as I know there is no example of
    an antigen which T cells do not recognize.

L. WASHINGTON: What is the situation in nude mice which have no T cells?

R. GERSHON: They make a very poor immune response consisting mainly of IgM antibodies. They are easily rendered tolerant. There is no switch from IgM to IgG. They do not make high affinity antibodies. Their response is much like that of the shark which also does not have T cells. There certainly is a T-independent response. Nobody disagrees with that. The point is that most of the important mammalian immune responses are T-dependent and T regulated. The nude mouse makes a response to SIII which is identical to a normal mouse But if you remove some T cells from a normal mouse his response to SIII is markedly augmented. So this augmentation is in a sense dependent upon T-cell control.

G.Schiffman:I would like to offer one word of caution about translating all of this mouse data to humans. In carrying out studies on pneumococcal vaccines, we found that some humans make a perfectly good IgG response to type III polysaccharide while others make a poor response. Furthermore, in infants the response is not as long lasting as it is in adults. Thus, even among humans there is a marked variation in the immune response to these antigens. I really do not think studies on mice can be directly extrapolated to the human.

R. GERSHON: I am not so sure about that. Of course, in the most detailed sense nothing should be extrapolated on a one to one basis. One should not extrapolate the response of a Balb/c mouse to a CBA mouse because there are very definite differences. It has for example, been shown that the response of mice to Type II pneumococcal polysaccharide has a T cell component, and one can obtain delayed hypersensitivity even to this antigen. Thus, you cannot even extrapolate from Type III to Type II pneumococcal polysaccharides. These things certainly are not absolute. However, even in humans antibodies against polysaccharides are often of the IgM class. Those that are IgG tend to be of low affinity. Most important T-cell dependent antibodies are those of high affinity. So that the story, while not permitting a simple one to one comparison of man and mouse, is still most impressive in terms of basic similarities.

SUPPRESSOR T CELLS IN IMMUNODEFICIENCY

Thomas A. Waldmann, S. Broder, M. Durm,
M. Blackman and B. Meade

Metabolism Branch, National Cancer Institute,
National Institutes of Health, Bethesda, Maryland

INTRODUCTION

The immunodeficiency diseases in man comprise an array of disorders which have been of great interest because they provide insights into the normal function of the immunologic system. The analysis of these disorders taken in conjunction with studies of experimental animal models have led to a greater understanding of the complex pathways of cellular differentiation, cellular interaction and cellular bio-synthesis that together are essential for the normal immune response. A general scheme of lymphoid cell function is shown graphically in Figure 1. There is now ample evidence that cells destined to subserve immunological functions arise from primitive stem cells located in the bone marrow. Such cells migrate to central lymphoid organs where under appropriate inductive influences they differentiate into cells that can interact with antigens and become effectors of the immune system. One route of this migration is through the thymus. At this site stem cells differentiate into T lymphocytes or T cells, which give rise to populations of cells that take part in cellular immune reactions. The development of antibody producing plasma cells can also be considered a discontinuous developmental process which can be divided conveniently into two stages. The first stage involves the primary differentiation of stem cells into immunocompetent B lymphocytes or B cells without the requirement of exogenous antigenic stimulation, but with the cooperation of a central lymphoid organ such as the bursa of Fabricius in birds, and its yet undefined equivalent in man.

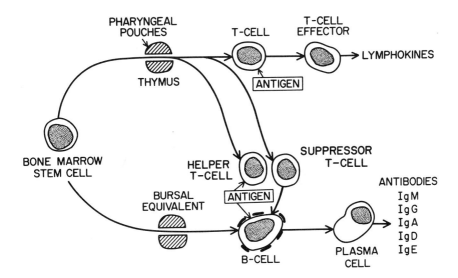

Figure 1. Scheme of cellular differentiation, cellular interaction and cellular biosynthesis required for specific immune response.

B cells can be identified in the peripheral blood as lymphocytes with surface membrane bound immunoglobulins in high
density. The membrane bound immunoglobulins are apparently
receptors through which antigens are recognized. The union
of appropriately presented antigen and membrane receptor
antibody trigger second stage events which include B-cell
proliferation and terminal differentiation into antibody
secreting plasma cells. This process of B-cell maturation
can also be stimulated by certain lectins including pokeweed
mitogen in man. All or most B cells appear to have cell
surface receptors for this mitogen by which they can be
triggered into terminal differentiation and immunoglobulin
synthesis.

The T and B-cell pathways of cellular differentiation
intersect in the course of the normal immune response.
Specifically, many antigens require the presence of both T
and B cells to induce a full circulating antibody response.
For these antigens the T cells serve as helper cells,
whereas B cells mature into the antibody synthesizing cells.
More recently, it has been recognized that certain T cells
may act as regulators of B-cell maturation and inhibit this
process. There is ample evidence for both antigen and
carrier specific as well as non-specific T-cell regulatory
or suppressor effects on antibody production (1-7).

The immunodeficiency diseases of man associated with
hypogammaglobulinemia have different disorders with defects
at distinct positions in the developmental sequence of
immunoglobulin producing cells. For example, patients with
severe combined immunodeficiency disease have a defect in
the stem cell precursors of immunocompetent cells. The
majority of patients with infantile X-linked agammaglobulinemia appear to have a defect in the differentiation
of these stem cells into B lymphocytes. Thus, patients
with X-linked agammaglobulinemia are usually quite deficient
in B lymphocytes bearing easily demonstrable membrane-bound
immunoglobulins (8-10). In contrast, many patients with
common variable immunodeficiency have normal percentages of
circulating B lymphocytes (8-11). Nevertheless, these
patients are unable to produce normal quantities of immunoglobulin. Similarly, most patients with isolated IgA
deficiency have normal proportions of IgA bearing B lymphocytes yet are unable to produce normal amounts of circulating
or secretory IgA (8,10,12). These observations led to the

view that patients with common variable immunodeficiency and
those with isolated IgA deficiency have a defect in the
terminal differentiation of B lymphocytes into mature immunoglobulin synthesizing and secreting cells.

    To analyze this defect, we developed a technique for the
study of the terminal differentiation of B lymphocytes
in vitro. This technique is of value in defining the nature
of this critical process and in defining the defects in
patients with immunodeficiency disorders. With the use of
this technique we found that lymphocytes from normal controls
synthesize each of the major classes of immunoglobulins
in vitro. In contrast, patients with common variable hypogammaglobulinemia fail to synthesize significant quantities
of any class of immunoglobulins. To determine whether the
failure of lymphocyte immunoglobulin synthesis by these
patients is due solely to an intrinsic defect in the maturation of their B lymphocytes or whether it could be due to
the presence of suppressor cells, we used procedures in which
lymphocytes of patients were co-cultured with normal lymphocytes. We were able to demonstrate in these co-culture
experiments that a large subset of the patients with common
variable immunodeficiency (7) or those with the syndrome of
thymoma and hypogammaglobulinemia have circulating suppressor
T cells which inhibit B-cell maturation and immunoglobulin
synthesis.

MATERIALS AND METHODS

    To study the terminal differentiation of lymphocytes,
exhaustively washed peripheral blood lymphocytes were
cultured *in vitro* in the presence or absence of the B-cell
mitogen, pokeweed mitogen. The immunoglobulin produced and
secreted by such cells after seven days was then measured
by sensitive double antibody radioimmunoassay techniques
specific for IgM, IgG or IgA. In this technique, supernatant
cells were obtained from 20 to 50 ml of heparinized blood
sedimented at 37°C. In order to remove all human serum
proteins, the cells were washed 12 times with balanced salt
solution containing 5% heat inactivated fetal calf serum.
Two million lymphocytes per ml were then incubated at 37°C in

5% CO_2 in loosely capped vials in the presence or absence
of pokeweed mitogen using RPMI 1640 media supplemented with
glutamine, penicillin, streptomycin and 10% fetal calf serum.
At the termination of the culture period, the tubes were
centrifuged at 2500 rpm (1200 g) for 10 minutes. The amount
of IgG, IgA and IgM synthesized and secreted into the culture
media was then determined by double antibody radioimmuno-
assays. The techniques for the production of the antisera,
defining their specificity and the performance of the radioimmunoassay were essentially identical to those previously
described for the double antibody radioimmunoassay of IgE
(13).

    In a number of studies, aliquots of cells obtained on
the seventh day of culture were assayed for cytoplasmic
immunoglobulin molecules by direct and indirect staining
using fluorescein labelled antibodies. Purified T cells were
prepared by spontaneous sheep cell rosette techniques
combined with density centrifugation (14). The T-cell
preparations were shown to contain less than 1% contamination
of B cells as assayed by cell surface immunofluorescence and
less than 1% macrophages as defined using a stain for non-
specific esterase (15).

EXPERIMENTAL RESULTS AND DISCUSSION

    Peripheral blood lymphocytes from normal individuals
synthesize and secrete modest quantities of immunoglobulins
when cultured in the absence of pokeweed mitogen (Table I).
In these studies the geometric mean synthetic rates of IgG,
IgA and IgM synthesis were 199, 207 and 586 ng per 2×10^6
lymphocytes respectively over the seven day culture period.
Immunoglobulin production by lymphocytes was markedly stimulated when pokeweed mitogen was added at the initiation of
the culture. The geometric mean synthetic rates for IgG,
IgA and IgM were 1625 ng, 1270 ng and 4910 ng per 2×10^6
lymphocytes respectively over the seven day culture period.
This represents a six to over eight-fold stimulation of
immunoglobulin synthesis in the presence of pokeweed mitogen
as compared to incubation in medium containing fetal calf
serum alone. An analysis of the time course of synthesis and

release of immunoglobulin molecules by lymphocytes in the presence of pokeweed mitogen indicated there was very little synthesis and release of immunoglobulin by lymphocytes during the first three to four days of culture. However, after this time the concentrations of immunoglobulin detectable in the culture medium increased rapidly, indicating maturation of non-immunoglobulin secreting B cells into immunoglobulin synthesizing and secreting cells.

TABLE I

Immunoglobulin Biosynthesis
by Peripheral Blood Lymphocytes

	Amount of Ig Synthesized		
	IgM[*] (ng)	IgA (ng)	IgG (ng)
Without PWM[†]	586	207	199
With PWM	4910	1270	1625
Ratio $\frac{\text{With PWM}}{\text{Without PWM}}$	8.4	6.1	8.2

[*] *Value presented as geometric mean of immunoglobulin synthesized in nanograms for a seven day culture of 2×10^6 normal lymphocytes.*

[†] *PWM - Pokeweed Mitogen*

The immunoglobulin synthetic process could be inhibited by at least 90% by irradiation of the cells with 2000 R or by the addition of puromycin (5×10^{-4}M), actinomycin D (10 µg/ml), mitomycin C (25 µg/ml), or cytosine arabinoside (2×10^{-4}M) to the culture medium. These studies taken in conjunction with the time course studies suggest that a critical mitosis is required before a major increase in lymphocyte immunoglobulin synthesis is possible following exposure of these cells to pokeweed mitogen.

In contrast to the stimulatory effect of pokeweed mitogen, the addition of the mitogens phytohemagglutinin, staphylococcal filtrate, or concanavalin A to the cultures of normal lymphocytes inhibited B-cell maturation and immunoglobulin synthesis. That is, when phytohemagglutinin (1 µg/ml), staphylococcal filtrate or concanavalin A (20 µg/ml) was added to cultures of normal lymphocytes in optimal mitogenic doses, pokeweed mitogen induced B-cell maturation and immunoglobulin synthesis were depressed to less than 16 percent of normal (Table II). Appropriate control studies were performed to demonstrate that this suppression was not due to either a cytotoxic effect of these mitogens on lymphocytes or to interference with the radioimmunoassay procedure for immunoglobulin molecules. Preliminary studies suggest that two mechanisms are of significance in this inhibitory process. The first mechanism is a direct inhibitory action of these soluble mitogens on B cells. It has been previously shown by others in the mouse and man that B cells have as many receptors for phytohemagglutinin and concanavalin A as do T cells (16,17). In preliminary studies using the present lymphocyte immunoglobulin biosynthesis procedure we have shown that concanavalin A and phytohemagglutinin inhibit the immunoglobulin synthesis of purified B cells. These studies suggest that these agents in soluble form may act to interfere with immunoglobulin production by interacting directly with the receptors for these mitogens on B cells leading to an inhibitory signal to these cells. A second mechanism for the inhibitory action of these mitogens is suggested by the work of Rich and Pierce (5) and Dutton (4). These workers have presented evidence that a subset of T cells can be activated by concanavalin A to non-specifically suppress antibody production by B cells. We have preliminary evidence supporting these observations. In these studies lymphocytes pulsed with concanavalin A for an 18-hour period inhibited immunoglobulin synthesis by untreated lymphocytes when they were co-cultured with them in the presence of pokeweed mitogen. These observations support the view that activated suppressor T cells or their products can act as non-specific inhibitory regulators of B-cell maturation and immunoglobulin synthesis.

TABLE II

Effect of "T" Cell Mitogens on Immunoglobulin Synthesis by Pokeweed Mitogen Stimulated Lymphocytes

	Percent Inhibition of Immunoglobulin Biosynthesis		
	IgM (%)	IgA (%)	IgG (%)
Concanavalin A (20 μg/ml)	98	95	94
Phytohemagglutinin (1 μg/ml)	88	96	84
Staph-Filtrate	97	95	93

The technique for the study of *in vitro* immunoglobulin biosynthesis and secretion was applied to the study of the peripheral blood lymphocytes from 18 patients with common variable hypogammaglobulinemia. The lymphocytes of 18 patients with this disorder studied were not able to make significant quantities of IgG, IgA or IgM *in vitro* in the presence or absence of pokeweed mitogen. There was also no evidence of lymphocyte immunoglobulin synthesis following culture with pokeweed mitogen as assessed by cytoplasmic immunofluorescence in 10 of the 11 patients studies.

Following culture the lymphocytes of the remaining patient had IgM and IgG in the cytoplasm as demonstrated by indirect staining using fluorescein labelled antibodies but did not have immunoglobulin detectable in the culture medium. This patient may have had a defect in immunoglobulin secretion comparable to that observed in patients studied by Choi, Bigger and Good (18) and Geha and coworkers (19). The remaining patients appear to have a disorder in the differentiation of B cells into cells which can synthesize immunoglobulin molecules.

To determine whether the failure of lymphocyte immunoglobulin synthesis by these patients with hypogammaglobulinemia was due solely to an intrinsic defect in the maturation of their B lymphocytes or whether it could be due to the presence of suppressor cells, the lymphocytes of patients with common variable hypogammaglobulinemia were co-cultured with lymphocytes from normal individuals. In these studies, one million lymphocytes from the patient were cultured together with one million normal lymphocytes in the presence of pokeweed mitogen. All other culture conditions were kept constant. The synthesis of immunoglobulins by the cells of the two subjects in co-culture was related to the sum of the expected contribution by each lymphocyte population using the following assumptions and formulae: If 2×10^6 lymphocytes from patient A synthesized α ng of Ig and if 2×10^6 lymphocytes from patient B synthesized β ng of Ig when cultured alone, then if the cells of A and B in co-culture do not stimulate or inhibit each other, 10^6 A lymphocyte and 10^6 B lymphocyte would be expected to synthesize $\frac{1}{2}(\alpha + \beta)$ nanograms of Ig when co-cultured. If the actual observed Ig synthesis in co-culture of cells from A and B is X, the fraction of the expected synthesis would be:

$$\frac{X}{\frac{1}{2}(\alpha + \beta)}$$

and the percent inhibition can be calculated from the expression:

$$\left\{1 - \frac{X}{\frac{1}{2}(\alpha + \beta)}\right\} \times 100.$$

Using this mode of analysis, the synthesis of immunoglobulins by normal cells was reduced by a factor of 75-100% when incubated with lymphocytes from 9 of the 13 hypogammaglobulinemic patients studied. All classes of immunoglobulins were affected. A typical study is shown in Figure 2. It can be seen that the lymphocytes from the normal individual

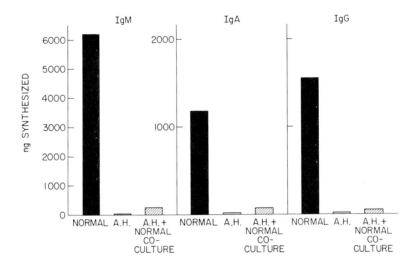

Figure 2. Inhibition of IgM, IgA and IgG synthesis
by normal lymphocytes when co-cultured with lymphocytes from a patient A.H. with common variable
hypogammaglobulinemia. The lymphocytes from the
normal individual synthesized from 1200 to over
6000 ng of the three major immunoglobulin
classes when cultured with pokeweed mitogen
alone. The synthesis of immunoglobulins by these
control cells was suppressed by a factor of over
90 percent when they were co-cultured with the
lymphocytes of patient A.H.

synthesized from 1200 to over 6000 ng of IgA, IgG and IgM
when cultured alone. The lymphocytes from AH with common
variable hypogammaglobulinemia did not synthesize significant quantities of any of the immunoglobulin classes. When
the cells of AH were cultured with those of the control, the
synthesis of Ig by the control cells was suppressed by a
factor of over 90%. When the cells from the hypogammaglobulinemic donor were irradiated with 6000 R or heated to 56°C
for 30 minutes before initiation of the co-culture experiments, no inhibition of synthesis was observed. Thus,
viable cells appear to be required for the observed suppression. To define the nature of the suppressing cell from
hypogammaglobulinemic patients, T cells free of B cells and
macrophages from patients with this disorder were isolated
from peripheral blood using a sheep cell rosette technique
and were used in co-culture experiments. Immunoglobulin
synthesis by normal lymphocytes stimulated by pokeweed
mitogen was markedly reduced when cultured with T cells from
patients with common variable hypogammaglobulinemia. Thus,
the synthesis of the major immunoglobulin classes by normal
lymphocytes was reduced by a factor of 85-100% when co-
cultured with T cells from patients with common variable
hypogammaglobulinemia.

A series of control studies was designed to determine
if the cellular suppression process was a specific property
of cells from patients with common variable hypogammaglobulinemia. It was found that co-culture of lymphocytes from
unrelated normal individuals did not result in significant
inhibition of immunoglobulin synthesis. Thus, the IgG, IgM
and IgA synthesized in co-culture by the lymphocytes of
20 pairs of unrelated normal donors gave mean values between
93 and 106% of the expected sum of the immunoglobulins
synthesized by the two individuals cultured separately.
Similarly, incubation of normal lymphocytes with lymphocytes
from patients with isolated IgA deficiency or the Sézary
syndrome, a T-cell leukemia, did not inhibit immunoglobulin
synthesis. Finally, there was no inhibition of immunoglobulin synthesis by the lymphocytes of seven normal individuals when they were co-cultured with isolated T cells from
unrelated normals. These studies indicate that the ability
of cells of one individual to inhibit immunoglobulin biosynthesis by cells from another is not a non-specific
phenomenon but is a special feature of the patients with
common variable hypogammaglobulinemia.

We have investigated the capacity of partially purified peripheral blood B lymphocytes from a patient with common variable hypogammaglobulinemia to synthesize immunoglobulins. These B lymphocytes were partially depleted of T cells by sheep cell rosetting techniques. The unseparated lymphocytes from the patient studied showed no immunoglobulin synthesis *in vitro* and suppressed the immunoglobulin synthesis by normal lymphocytes by greater than 90%. In contrast, the B-cell enriched, T-cell depleted fraction from this patient did not suppress the immunoglobulin biosynthesis by normal lymphocytes. In addition, these T-cell depleted lymphocytes synthesized 1480 ng of IgM/2 × 10^6 when cultured with poke-weed mitogen *in vitro*. These studies suggest that, in a significant subset of patients with common variable hypo-gammaglobulinemia, the defect is caused or perpetuated by an abnormality of regulatory, suppressor T cells which act to inhibit B-cell maturation and antibody synthesis. That is, in this subset the patients do not appear to have an intrin-sic defect in the maturation of their B lymphocytes but rather have an abnormal number or an abnormally activated set of suppressor T cells.

Certain patients with a thymoma or with multiple myeloma have hypogammaglobulinemia and an increased incidence of infections. When the immunoglobulin biosynthesis technique was applied to the study of lymphocytes from two patients with thymoma and hypogammaglobulinemia, a pattern similar to that observed with common variable hypogammaglobulinemia was obtained. That is, the lymphocytes from these two patients with hypogammaglobulinemia and thymoma studied, synthesized less than 100 ng of each class of immunoglobulin during the study period. When lymphocytes from these patients were co-cultured with normal lymphocytes and pokeweed mitogen, the synthesis of immunoglobulin by the normal lymphocytes was depressed by a factor of 66-97%. Incubation of the normal lymphocytes with purified T cells of the patients with thymoma and hypogammaglobulinemia resulted in suppression of immunoglobulin synthesis by a factor of 73-100%. Thus, suppressor T cells may play a role in the pathogenesis of hypogammaglobulinemia and defective antibody production observed in the patients with thymoma and hypogamma-globulinemia studied.

Patients with multiple myeloma have a significant reduction in *in vivo* polyclonal immunoglobulin synthesis (20)

and in the serum levels of polyclonal immunoglobulin (21) as
well as in the percentage of circulating lymphocytes that
have normal surface immunoglobulins (22). Such patients have
a reduced capacity to synthesize antibody in response to
antigenic challenge and have an increased incidence of
infections with highly pathogenic encapsulated bacteria. We
have applied the *in vitro* immunoglobulin biosynthesis
measurement to the study of peripheral blood lymphocytes from
22 patients with myeloma. The lymphocytes of the patients
studied showed profound depression of polyclonal (non-
paraprotein class) immunoglobulin production. Thus, the
geometric mean polyclonal immunoglobulin synthetic rates
were 458 ng for IgM, 321 ng for IgA and 216 ng for IgG per
two million lymphocytes in the presence of pokeweed mitogen.
These mean values are approximately 10% of the mean values of
normal individuals. Peripheral blood lymphocytes from three
of the six patients with myeloma tested, suppressed the polyclonal immunoglobulin synthesis of normal lymphocytes in co-
culture. Suppression generally ranged from 75–100%.
However, in contrast to the observations in patients with
common variable hypogammaglobulinemia or with thymoma and
hypogammaglobulinemia, this suppression was not observed
when purified T lymphocytes from patients with myeloma were
co-cultured with normal lymphocytes. These observations
suggest that one mechanism for the humoral immunodeficiency
observed in myeloma patients is a block of polyclonal lymphocyte maturation by suppressor cells. T cells alone do
not appear to mediate this suppression.

We next applied the *in vitro* lymphocyte immunoglobulin
biosynthesis technique to the study of patients with the
immunodeficiency syndrome, isolated IgA deficiency.
Virtually all of these patients with absence of IgA from
their serum and secretions had normal numbers of circulating
IgA bearing B lymphocytes. In the *in vitro* culture system,
lymphocytes of these patients secreted virtually no IgA into
the medium. However, in contrast to the lymphocytes of
patients with common variable hypogammaglobulinemia, eight
of nine such patients studied had cells with IgA in their
cytoplasm as assessed by cytoplasmic immunofluorescent
studies following seven days of *in vitro* culture in the
presence of pokeweed mitogen. These studies suggest that at
least limited IgA synthesis is possible in response to pokeweed mitogen in such patients but that secretion of IgA by
these cells is abnormal. In general, such patients did not
have circulating or cellular inhibitors of B-cell maturation

nor could they be made to synthesize and secrete IgA into the
media using a variety of techniques. There was one interest-
ing exception to this latter generalization. In this patient
there was a severe defect in thymic function as well as the
defect in IgA production. The cells of this patient did not
make significant quantities of IgA when cultured with pokeweed mitogen alone. However, when T cells from a particular
patient with the small cell variety of the Sézary syndrome
which did not in themselves synthesize IgA were added to the
culture system, the lymphocytes of the patient with thymic
and IgA deficiencies synthesized over 30,000 ng of IgA per
1×10^6 lymphocytes in culture. This observation supports
the view that an interaction of T and B cells might be
required for the differentiation of appropriate B cells into
IgA synthesizing and secreting cells.

SUMMARY

The physiological and pathophysiological factors
regulating immunoglobulin synthesis and the role of suppressor and helper T cells in this process were analyzed using a
technique which permits the study of the terminal differentiation of B lymphocytes into immunoglobulin synthesizing and
secreting cells. The peripheral blood lymphocytes from
normal individuals synthesized 4910 ng of IgM, 1270 ng of
IgA and 1625 ng of IgG/2×10^6 cells when cultured for seven
days in the presence of pokeweed mitogen. The addition of
mitogens phytohemagglutinin, staphylococcal filtrate or
concanavalin A to the media with normal lymphocytes prevented
B-cell maturation and immunoglobulin synthesis. Evidence
supporting two mechanisms for this immunosuppression are
presented. In the first mechanism, direct interaction of
these mitogens with mitogen receptors on B cells results in
suppression of B-cell differentiation into immunoglobulin
synthesizing and secreting cells. In the second mechanism
suppressor T cells are activated and in turn prevent B-cell
maturation.

The lymphocytes from the 18 patients with common
variable immunodeficiency and two patients with thymoma and
hypogammaglobulinemia studied did not synthesize and secrete

significant quantities of any major class of immunoglobulin *in vitro* in the presence of pokeweed mitogen during the seven day culture period. In addition, when the lymphocytes from nine of the 13 patients with common variable immunodeficiency or from the two patients with thymoma and hypogammaglobulinemia studied were incubated with normal lymphocytes and pokeweed mitogen, the synthesis and secretion of immunoglobulin by normal cells was inhibited. T cells were shown to mediate the inhibition in both the patients with common variable immunodeficiency and those with thymoma and hypogammaglobulinemia. These observations suggest that, in some patients, the disease common variable hypogammaglobulinemia and the syndrome thymoma and hypogammaglobulinemia may be caused or perpetuated by an abnormality of regulatory T cells which act to suppress B cell maturation and antibody production. In other studies, polyclonal immunoglobulin synthesis was reduced when lymphocytes from patients with multiple myeloma were studied using this assay. Circulatory suppressor cells, other than T cells, were shown to be a potential factor in the reduced polyclonal immunoglobulin synthesis of these patients with myeloma.

Patients with isolated IgA deficiency produced IgA following incubation *in vitro* with pokeweed mitogen as demonstrated by cytoplasmic immunofluorescent studies. However, virtually no IgA was demonstrable in the medium. This suggests that such patients either have a quantitative defect in the amount of IgA they can synthesize or have a defect in the secretion of synthesized IgA from their cells.

REFERENCES

1. Gershon, R.K., Contempory Topics in Immunobiol., *3*: 1, 1974.

2. Baker, P.J., Stashak, P.W., Amsbaugh, D.F., Prescott, B. and Barth, R.F., J. Immunol., *105*: 1581, 1970.

3. Okumura, K. and Tada, T., J. Immunol., *106*: 1019, 1971.

4. Dutton, R.W., J. Exp. Med., *138:* 1496, 1973.

5. Rich, R.R. and Pierce, C.W., J. Exp. Med., *137*: 649, 1973.

6. Jacobson, E.B., Herzenberg, L.A., Riblet, R. and Herzenberg, L.A., J. Exp. Med., *135*: 1163, 1972.

7. Waldmann, T.A., Broder, S., Blaese, R.M., Durm, M., Blackman, M. and Strober, W., Lancet, *2*: 609, 1974.

8. Grey, H.M., Rabellino, E. and Pirofsky, B., J. Clin. Invest., *50*: 2368, 1971.

9. Preud'homme, J.L. and Seligmann, M., Lancet, *1*: 442, 1972.

10. Gajl-Peczalska, K.H., Park, B.H., Biggar, W.D. and Good, R.A., J. Clin. Invest., *52*: 919, 1973.

11. Cooper, M.D., Lawton, A.R. and Bockman, D.E., Lancet, *2*: 791, 1971.

12. Lawton, A.R., Royal, S.A., Self, K.S. and Cooper, M.D., J. Lab. Clin. Med., *80*: 26, 1972.

13. Waldmann, T.A., Polmar, S.H., Balestra, S.T., Jost, M.C., Bruce, R.M. and Terry, W.D., J. Immunol., *109*: 304, 1972

14. Wybran, J., Chantler, S. and Fudenberg, H.H., Lancet, *1*: 126, 1973.

15. Yam, L.T., Li, C.Y. and Crosby, W.H., Am. J. Clin. Path., *55*: 283, 1971.

16. Stobo, J.D., Rosenthal, A.S. and Paul, W.E., J. Immunol., *108*: 1, 1972.

17. Boldt, D.H., MacDermott, R.P. and Jorolan, E.P., J. Immunol., In Press.

18. Choi, Y.S., Biggar, W.D. and Good, R.A., Lancet, *1*: 1149, 1972.

19. Geha, R.S., Schneeberger, E., Merler, E. and Rosen, F.S., New Eng. J. Med., *291*: 1, 1974.

20. Waldmann, T.A. and Strober, W., Prog. Allergy, *13*: 1, 1969.

21. Fahey, J.L., Scoggins, R., Utz, J.P. and Szwed, C.F.,
     Am. J. Med., *35*: 698, 1963.

22. Lindström, F.D., Hardy, W.R., Eberle, B.J. and
     Williams, R.C., Jr., Ann. Intern. Med., *78*: 837, 1973.

DISCUSSION FOLLOWING PRESENTATION

by DR. THOMAS A. WALDMANN

G. SISKIND: Have you studied any classical Bruton's-type
    agammaglobulinemia patients? Do they have detectable
    suppressor activity?

T. WALDMANN: We have tried to study a number of patients
    other than the common variable immune deficiency group.
    We have studied severe combined immunodeficiency disease
    and they do not have suppressor cells. With regard to
    the x-linked agammaglobulinemia patients we have only
    had an opportunity to study those rare patients who have
    immunoglobulin on their B cells. These patients do not
    have suppressor cells. We have not had an opportunity
    to study classical Bruton's-type agammaglobulinemia
    patients. I would not be surprised if one were to see,
    as a secondary event, suppressor cells in these indivi-
    duals. The studies of Jacobson and Herzenberg were
    referred to earlier. The phenomenon of allotype
    suppression which they studied was not initiated by
    suppressor T cells but by injection of antibody to an
    allotype. However, allotype suppression appears to be
    perpetuated by the action of suppressor T cells. That
    is, the suppressor T cells act as a secondary event to
    maintain allotype suppression. Studies in our labora-
    tory on bursectomized birds also suggest that suppressor
    T cells become evident and serve to perpetuate the
    depression of immune responsiveness as a secondary
    event.

M. DeSOUSA: At what time can you add the putative suppressor
    T cells to a culture already stimulated by pokeweed
    mitogen and still observe suppression?

T. WALDMANN: This is a question to which we have addressed
ourselves a number of times. Experimentally it has some
difficulties since it requires a rewashing of the cells.
We have done the experiment at 24 hours and we find we
can still get suppression although to a reduced extent.
Later than 24 hours we have not seen suppression, however, we have not carried out the experiment a sufficient
number of times to be certain. I should warn you that
the suppressor T cells are somewhat evanescent in tissue
culture systems. Thus, you must start your pokeweed
study with one individual and then come in with freshly
prepared T cells at another time. In summary, both in
terms of our pulsing studies with concanavalin-A and with
suppressor T cells one can obtain suppression at 24 hours
however, it is already much reduced. After that I do
not think you can get suppression. These cells do not
suppress when given on the seventh day of culture or
when given to B-cell cultured lines making immunoglobulin. Consequently, we do not feel that this is a
procedure which turns off fully differentiated immunoglobulin secreting cells. It is certainly not the
result of a cytotoxic effect of the suppressor cells.

R. GERSHON: I do not know if this is the appropriate place
to ask this question as it might be a bit controversial.
In your first slide you showed cells going to a bursal
equivalent and then coming out. In the second slide
the cells were still going through a bursal equivalent
and now a suppressor T cell is interacting with them.
I wonder if one can combine your results and those of
Mike Blaese and the claim by Droge, for which I find the
evidence quite convincing, that in the chicken the
suppressor T cell comes from the bursa. Is it not
possible that in mammals and humans a portion of the
bursal equivalent is actually the thymus?

T. WALDMANN: I do not really think our results address this
issue. Mike Blaese bursectomized birds have suppressor
T cells. He studies an infectious agammaglobulinemia
in which he transplants normal marrow with or without
added marrow from bursectomized birds to irradiated
intact animals. What you see is immunoglobulin production initially, followed by termination of immunoglobulin synthesis when you have given bursectomized
bird marrow in addition to the normal marrow. I, and I

believe he, interpret this data as showing the presence of suppressor T cells even in birds which were bursectomized at hatching.

R. GERSHON: Since the above findings are related to the bursa, and if Droge is correct and there is a bursa dependent T-cell population which has suppressor activity, then the possibility I raised is worth considering. Then there is the other side of the story. If you do find suppressor function I would predict that you will find a helper function as the two seem to travel hand-in-hand.

T. WALDMANN: Not everyone of course views the suppressor and helper cells as identical. I know you hold that opinion very strongly. But certainly there are groups such as Melman and Scher who feel that they may be able to separate helper from suppressor T-cell activity by use of histimine-albumin-sepharose columns. We are, therefore, keeping an open mind on this question. With our patients we are using such columns in an effort to remove suppressor T-cell activity. Clearly this is an important question and I feel a still open one.

R. GOOD: These are certainly very beautiful results. When studying cultures after five to seven days what loss of cells do you see during culture? What is the ratio of the number of cells you start with to the number you have left at the end of the culture period?

T. WALDMANN: In general, when two million cells from agammaglobulinemia patients are cultured alone we get between half and one million cells left in the culture at the end of seven days.   In the co-culture experiments we find between 25 and 75% of the cells placed initially in culture still viable at the end of the culture period. We do not feel that we have cytotoxic lymphocyte type activity going on. In terms of human peripheral blood cultures we are still getting considerable synthesis beyond seven days. This is in sharp contrast to the experience of many people who work with mouse spleen where if you go three or four days you are getting all of the IgM production.

With human peripheral blood cultures you can go as long
as 14 days and instead of having 4,000 ng of IgM, you
have 16,000 to 20,000 ng of IgM produced. The cells are
still viable. Our own feeling in terms of the number of
viable cells in the culture is that it is not effected
by whether you use normal cells or co-cultures of normal
cells and agammaglobulinemic cells. I do not feel that
we have anything like the action of a cytotoxic lymphocyte. There are significant numbers of cells in culture
at the end of the experiment.

GREENBLATT: Have you attempted to titrate the cells in the
common variable immune deficiency syndrome? That is,
have you mixed a million normal cells with various
numbers of common variable immune deficiency cells?

T. WALDMANN: We really have not. Each time we have
attempted that type of study on a new patient it has
turned out to be one of those individuals who does not
suppress. Thus, we have never done such a titration
with suppressor T cells.

SCHWARTZ: Have you looked at suppressor effect on
unstimulated cell populations? That is, on cultures
that did not receive pokeweed mitogen?

T. WALDMANN: The cells are in fact stimulated by the
presence of fetal calf serum in the culture medium even
if you do not add pokeweed mitogen. If you culture lymphocytes in the absence of fetal calf serum, or in poor
quality fetal calf serum, then you do not get immunoglobulin synthesis and release. However, in the presence
of fetal calf serum, cultures at the seventh day
synthesize between 200 and 500 ng of the three immunoglobulin classes which we have studied. By the 21st
day you are getting really significant immunoglobulin
concentrations in the supernates of such cultures.
When suppressor cells from common variable immunodeficiency patients are co-cultured with normal cells
in the presence of fetal calf serum they suppress this
"background" synthesis and release of immunoglobulin.
Thus, we do not need to have pokeweed mitogen in the
system to see complete suppression. It is not

competition for this mitogen which is involved.

S. LITWIN: We have been following a patient with immunoglobulin deficiency and red blood cell agenesis. The
red cell aplasia remitted after therapy with adrenal
corticoids. Is there any evidence for suppressors of
red cell precursors?

T. WALDMANN: I have thought about this. We are all aware of
the association of thymoma and pure red cell aplasia.
In about 20% of these patients the red cell aplasia
reverses upon removal of the thymoma. There is also
Sandy Krantz's work years ago. He concluded that there
is a circulating (perhaps IgG) inhibitor of red cell
precursors in the marrow. He treated such patients with
6-mercaptopurine with good results. We have not set up
systems involving culture of marrow even though my
research work started with studies on erythropoietin.
Thus, I really have no information on this possiblity.
We are studying very actively and getting some positive
results with T-T suppressor systems. But this is most
preliminary and we have not looked at the red cell at
all.

R. GERSHON: In answer to Dr. Litwin's question, in mice when
you elicit a chronic GVH you start out with most of the
increase in spleen weight being due to hematopoietic
cells, mainly myelobasts and erythroblasts. You see a
tremendous proliferation of these cells as a result of
the GVH. When the GVH enters a chronic phase the hematopoietic cells are then markedly depressed. It is
hard to rule out the possibility of a direct toxic event.
My own impression, from studying the slides, is that
there is a suppressive event occurring in chronic GVH.
There is a suppression of both polys and red cells.

ROLE OF SUPPRESSOR CELLS IN THE PATHOGENESIS
OF AUTOIMMUNITY IN NEW ZEALAND MICE

Alfred D. Steinberg, M.E. Gershwin, N.L. Gerber,
J.A. Hardin, D. Barthold, L.M. Parker, T.M. Chused

National Institutes of Health
Bethesda, Maryland

INTRODUCTION

New Zealand Black (NZB) mice and the hybrid (NZB/W) produced by crossing NZB mice with New Zealand White (NZW) mice spontaneously develop autoimmune phenomena mimicking those manifested by patients with systemic lupus erythematosus (SLE). These include antibodies to nucleic acids, erythrocytes and lymphoid cells as well as immune complex glomerulonephritis. A number of immunologic abnormalities in NZB and NZB/W mice have been reported from many laboratories around the world (1). These include premature responsiveness to immunization with sheep red blood cells (SRBC) and loss of induction and maintenance of tolerance to certain foreign protein antigens. Later in life these animals have impairment of many more immunologic functions including ability to mount normal cellular immune reactions and to respond to primary immunization with thymic dependent antigens.

During the course of cataloguing these various immuno-logic abnormalities, we undertook a series of experiments designed to develop an understanding of an orderly sequence of immunologic stages in the life of the NZB and NZB/W mice. We hoped thereby to determine whether or not some of the abnormalities were secondary to others, with the aim of simplifying the defects into some understandable scheme. In these studies we placed a major emphasis on regulation of the immune system. Early in life New Zealand mice appear to lose regulatory or suppressor cells. This is followed by the development of high titers of autoantibodies. Subsequently helper T-cell function is lost for both humoral and cellular immunity, and finally major autoimmune processes lead to death. We herein describe specific experiments which suggest that loss of suppressor function plays an important role in the pathogenesis of autoimmunity.

EXPERIMENTAL RESULTS

Studies with ATS and Polymeric Antigens.

Type III pneumococcal polysaccharide (SSSIII) does not appear to require helper T cells for the production of an antibody response. Baker pointed out that administration of an antiserum which inactivates mouse lymphocytes (ALS) at the time of immunization with SSSIII leads to an enhanced anti-body response to the SSSIII (2). This result suggested the existence of thymic derived regulatory or suppressor cells which normally serve to inhibit or regulate the antibody response to SSSIII. In the absence of such regulatory cells, the antibody response to SSSIII is enhanced. An alternative explanation might be that the ALS acted as a non-specific adjuvant. However, when thymocytes were given to mice one day after receiving SSSIII plus ALS, a marked degree of suppression of the antibody response to SSSIII was observed, suggesting that a non-specific adjuvant effect was not solely responsible. Rather, it appeared that by restoring the suppressor cells killed by the ALS a response similar to that following SSSIII alone was observed. A second population of enhancing cells was found in the peripheral blood. These studies suggest that the cellular regulation of the antibody response to what had previously appeared to be a "thymic independent" antigen is in fact complicated. At least two populations of cells appear to regulate the response through enhancing or suppressing action.

With the discovery that suppressor function could be studied by the administration of ALS as described above, we decided to study the response of NZB/W and control mice to the synthetic double stranded RNA polyinosinic·polycytidylic

acid (rI.rC) and anti-thymocyte serum (ATS) (3). The first
study confirmed with rI.rC the observations made with SSSIII
(Table I). With age NZB/W mice lost the ability to have the
anti-RNA response enchanced with ATS (Table II). These
studies suggested an age associated loss of immune regulatory
function. The study was complicated by the spontaneous
production of antibodies to RNA. This was circumvented by
studying the response to SSSIII to which New Zealand mice do
not spontaneously produce antibodies (4). We found an age
associated increase in the antibody response of NZB mice to
immunization with SSSIII (Table III). The increased response
of older NZB mice was significantly reduced by syngeneic
thymocytes from four week old donors, but not by cells from
older mice (Table IV).

Graft versus Host (GVH) Disease

     The apparent loss with age of suppressor cells was
further studied in the GVH system (5,6). The ability of
spleen cells from NZB/W mice to produce GVH varied with the
age of the donor NZB/W mice. Young and old NZB/W mice were
less able to mount a vigorous GVH response at a dose of
5×10^6 cells than were intermediate aged mice. Two
separate groups of experiments performed one year apart
produced the same general response curve with age (Table V).
Control C57BL/6 spleen cells did not show this rise and fall
in GVH activity during the first year of life (Table V).
C57BL/6 mice showed some reduction in spleen index (SI) at
24 months; however, significant GVH (SI > 1.30) was still
induced by cells from 24-month old C57BL/6 mice whereas 12-
month old NZB/W spleen cells were ineffective. The
reduction of GVH late in life in NZB/W mice was found to be
due to a loss of recirculating helper cells. The rise in
GVH activity in the first six months of life was the subject
of further investigation. Small numbers of spleen cells from
1½ month NZB/W mice suppressed the GVH response of 5×10^5
cells from 1½ month mice ($0.1 > P > 0.05$), but was highly
significant at 1×10^6 cells ($P < 0.001$).

     Thymocytes from NZB/W mice of different ages were mixed
with 5×10^6 spleen cells from 4½ month old NZB/W mice in an
attempt to determine when thymic regulatory function was lost.

TABLE I

Enhanced Antibody Response of BALB/c Mice
to rI·rC (100µg) in Aqueous Solution
when given with ATS*

Treatment	Anti-rI·rC Antibody Concentration†	
	Day 5	Day 8
None	<0.5	<0.5
rI·rC	2.8	2.6
rI·rC + NRS	2.7	1.8
rI·rC + ATS	13.8	8.1

* *NRS = Normal rabbit serum*
    ATS = Rabbit anti-mouse thymocyte serum
rI·rC = The double stranded RNA, polyinosinic
        polycytidylic acid

† *µg antigen bound per ml serum.*

One million thymocytes from mice aged one through four
months did not induce GVH (Table VII). The addition of
1×10^6 thymocytes from one month old NZB/W mice reduced the
GVH reaction induced by 5×10^6 spleen cells from $4\frac{1}{2}$ month
NZB/W mice from 1.75 to 1.29 ($P < 0.01$). There was a gradual
reduction with age in ability of this dose of thymocytes to
suppress the GVH induced by 5×10^6 spleen cells from

TABLE II

*Age-Dependent Loss in NZB/W Mice of ATS-Induced
Enhancement of the Antibody Response
to rI·rC (100 μg)*[*]

Age (months)	Treatment		Anti-rI·rC Antibody Concentration[†]	
	rI·rC	ATS	5 day	8 day
2	−	−	0.6	0.4
	+	−	2.1	0.5
	+	+	3.9	2.1
5	−	−	3.6	3.0
	+	−	4.2	3.6
	+	+	4.8	3.9
6	−	−	7.0	ND
	+	−	7.2	ND
	+	+	7.9	ND

[*] *rI·rC = the double stranded RNA, polyinosinic
polycytidylic acid.*

[†] *μg antigen bound per ml serum.*

TABLE III

*Antibody Response of Female NZB Mice
of Various Ages to Immunization
with 0.5 μg SSSIII**

Age (months)	PFC/Spleen	
	Geometric mean	Log_{10} ± S.E.M.
$1^{\dagger}$	2,160	3.33 ± 0.07
$1\frac{1}{2}$	3,647	3.56 ± 0.05§
3-4	6,500	3.81 ± 0.03$^{\Psi}$
6	10,369	4.02 ± 0.07$^{\Psi}$
9-11	11,390	4.06 ± 0.07$^{\downarrow}$

† *Three and one-half weeks of age.*

§ *P < 0.05 compared to next younger age.*

Ψ *P < 0.005 compared to next younger age.*

↓ *Not significantly different from next younger age.*

* *SSSIII = Type III pneumococcal polysaccharide*

$4\frac{1}{2}$ month NZB/W mice (Table VII). Increasing numbers of one
month thymocytes led to increased suppression which
approached a plateau between 2.5×10^6 thymocytes (Table VI).
In other experiments 1×10^6 thymocytes from one month
NZB/W mice were combined with varying numbers of spleen cells

TABLE IV

The Antibody Response to SSSIII[*] of Ten Month Old Female NZB Recipient Mice Receiving 50 × 10⁶ Cells from Different NZB Tissues

Donor Tissue		PFC/Spleen		
Organ	Age (months)	Geometric mean	Log_{10} ± S.E.M.	P value[†]
None		11,390	4.06 ± 0.07	
Thymus	1	6,459	3.81 ± 0.07	P < 0.01
Thymus	2	9,567	3.98 ± 0.18	NS[§]
Bone marrow	1	11,225	4.05 ± 0.06	NS
Spleen	1	10,960	4.04 ± 0.11	NS
Spleen	2	12,346	4.09 ± 0.03	NS

[*] SSSIII = Type III pneumococcal polysaccharide.

[†] All statistical comparisons are between the treated group and the group receiving no cells.

[§] NS, not significant P > 0.05.

TABLE V

Spleen Index on Day 9 of CEH/HEJ Mice Injected at Birth
with 5 × 10⁶ Spleen Cells from Female Mice of Different Ages

Strain	Age (months)	Spleen Index (Mean ± Standard Error of the Mean)
NZB/W	1	1.24* ± 0.18
	1½	1.41† ± 0.09
	2½	1.66 ± 0.11
	4½	1.75§ ± 0.04
	6	2.01§ ± 0.06
	9	1.50 ± 0.16
	12	1.19* ± 0.06
C57BL/6	1½	2.14⁺ ± 0.32
	5½	2.17⁺ ± 0.08
	12	1.99⁺ ± 0.15
	24	1.41 ± 0.40

* $P < 0.001$ compared with either 4½ or 6 month, Student's t-test.
† $P < 0.01$ compared with either 4½ or 6 month, Student's t-test.
§ Not significantly different.
⁺ Not significantly different.

49

TABLE VI

Reduction in Graft-vs-Host response of 5 × 10⁶ Spleen Cells from 4½ month NZB/W Mice by Syngeneic One Month Thymocytes and of 5 × 10⁶ Spleen Cells from Six Month Old NZB/W Mice by Syngeneic 1½ Month Old Spleen Cells

Number of Thymocytes Added	Suppression (percent)	Number of Spleen Cells Added	Suppression (percent)
1×10^5	5	1.25×10^5	4
5×10^5	38	5×10^5	30
10×10^5	62	10×10^5	55
25×10^5	74		
50×10^5	81		

TABLE VII

Graft-vs-Host Response to 1×10^6 NZB/W Thymocytes
of Different Ages, 5×10^6 Spleen Cells
from NZB/W Mice, and Combinations
of Thymocytes and Spleen Cells

Age of Donor Cell Population(s)		Spleen Index
Thymocytes (1×10^6) (months)	Spleen Cells (5×10^6) (months)	(Mean ± Standard Error of the Mean)
1	--	1.00 ± 0.08
2	--	1.04 ± 0.06
3	--	1.11 ± 0.06
4	--	1.12 ± 0.04
-	$4\frac{1}{2}$	1.75* ± 0.04
1	$4\frac{1}{2}$	1.29† ± 0.09
2	$4\frac{1}{2}$	1.34§ ± 0.10
3	$4\frac{1}{2}$	1.58* ± 0.10
4	$4\frac{1}{2}$	1.71* ± 0.16
-	12	1.19 ± 0.06
1	12	1.49Ψ ± 0.05
4	12	1.51Ψ ± 0.03

* *Not significantly different.*

† *$P < 0.01$ compared with $4\frac{1}{2}$ month spleen cells alone, Student's t-test.*

§ *$P < 0.05$ compared with $4\frac{1}{2}$ month spleen cells alone, Student's t-test.*

Ψ *$P < 0.05$ compared with 12 month spleen cells alone, Student's t-test.*

from $4\frac{1}{2}$ month NZB/W mice. Reducing the number of $4\frac{1}{2}$ month spleen cells from 5×10^6 to 2.5×10^6 led to a reduction in GVH, which was further reduced by the addition of one month thymocytes. One million $4\frac{1}{2}$ month spleen cells did not induce GVH. The addition of one month thymocytes did not increase the response.

Since lymphoid cells from one month old NZB/W mice have little GVH activity, but suppress the activity of syngeneic spleen cells capable of a vigorous GVH response, it remained a possibility that lymphoid cells from an NZB/W mouse with poor GVH reactivity would always lead to suppression. We, therefore, tested the ability of spleen cells from 12 month old mice, which do not induce GVH, to suppress the activity of six month old NZB/W spleen cells. When 1×10^6 spleen cells from 12 month old mice were mixed with 5×10^6 spleen cells from six month old mice no suppression was observed, whereas 1×10^6 spleen cells from $1\frac{1}{2}$ month old mice was suppressive.

It should be emphasized that thymocytes from three to four month old NZB/W mice are capable of acting as helper cells in collaboration with 12 month old spleen cells in the GVH reaction and in collaboration with three month old bone marrow cells in the antibody response to sheep erythrocytes. Therefore, the loss of suppressor function occurs at a time when helper function is still present. In fact, aliquots of the three and four month thymocyte preparations, which were unable to suppress the GVH response, acted as helper cells in the GVH and SRBC systems. These and other studies suggest (but do not prove) that distinct helper and suppressor populations are mediating the different functions.

Studies with Concanavalin A (Con A).

Con A is capable of inducing or activating suppressor activity *in vitro* (7,8). It has been found to depress both cellular and humoral immunity *in vitro* and *in vivo*. We, therefore, tried to increase tolerance to BGG in NZB/W mice with *in vivo* Con A treatment (9). This was of particular interest because loss of tolerance to ultracentrifuged bovine gamma globulin (BGG) in NZB/W mice seems to correlate with

loss of suppressor function. Two week old NZB/W mice were
made tolerant but rapidly escaped as had been found before
(1). When Con A treatment was given in addition to ultracentrifuged BGG, more prolonged tolerance was observed
(Figure 1). Four week old NZB/W mice were not made tolerant
to ultracentrifuged BGG. Treatment with Con A plus ultracentrifuged BGG led to transient tolerance to challenge with
BGG in adjuvant (Figure 2). The change in antibody titer
with time in four week old mice given Con A plus BGG was
similar to that of two week old mice given BGG only. These
studies suggest that Con A may be able to increase border-
line suppressor activity. They argue for a primary role of
suppressor cells in the loss of tolerance in NZB/W mice and
suggest the possibility of therapeutic intervention.

Thymic Factors.

Studies by Dauphinee and Talal (10) produced results
very similar to those observed in the GVH assay. They
utilized a system popularized by Gershon for study of the
proliferative response of NZB thymocytes in allogeneic
recipients (11). Two week old thymocytes from NZB mice had
normal proliferative responses, whereas eight week old
thymocytes were abnormal. Following the observation that
thymic hormone was reduced prematurely as NZB mice aged (12)
Dauphinee and co-workers studied the proliferative response
of the NZB cells with and without thymosin treatment (13).
Thymosin was able to correct the abnormality of older NZB
lymphoid cells.

Based upon these observations we have been studying the
effect of thymosin upon the natural history of New Zealand
mice. It appears that thymosin can improve some of the
immunologic defects of older NZB/W mice (14); however, non-
specific immune enhancers have also recently been found to
be effective (unpublished observations) leaving the question
of specificity open. More important, a large number of
NZB/W mice have been treated with thymosin in various
schedules starting at different ages. These studies have
not yielded dramatic therapeutic results. Either we were
not giving the proper material at the proper times or this
form of hormone therapy may not be as fruitful as was
originally hoped.

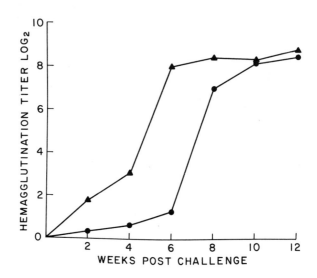

Figure 1. NZB/NZW (B/W) mice of both sexes were
treated with nothing or Con A starting at two
weeks of age and with ultracentrifuged bovine
gamma globulin (BGG) at 20 days of age and
challenged at 30 days of age with BGG in complete Freund's adjuvant (CFA). Mice receiving
Con A (closed circles) had a delayed escape
from tolerance compared with those receiving
ultracentrifuged BGG alone (closed triangles).

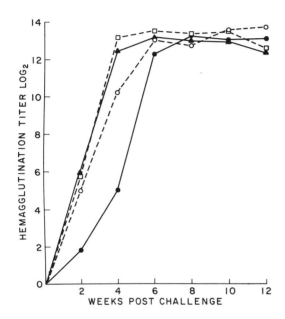

Figure 2. NZB/NZW (B/W) males were given ultracentrifuged BGG at 28 days of age (closed
circles) or Con A alone (open circles) or
neither (open squares). All mice were
challenged ten days later with BGG in CFA.
Mice receiving ultracentrifuged BGG plus
Con A had significantly lower antibody
titers two and four weeks post-challenge.

Thymic Grafting.

Cellular reconstitution experiments have proven to be somewhat more encouraging. Neonatal thymectomy leads to acceleration of the autoimmune disease of NZB/W mice. This acceleration was prevented by two week but not ten week syngeneic thymic grafts, suggesting that the younger thymuses have some regulatory influence whereas the older thymuses do not (15). This result led to therapy of NZB/W mice with two week old thymic grafts and thymocytes with only marginal success (16). It appeared that the therapy was having detrimental as well as desirable effects. The beneficial effects appeared to be eliminated by corticosteroid pretreatment of the thymus donors. Greater success has been obtained in the NZB mice. This was first reported by Allison, Playfair and co-workers (17). Although their actual data have not yet been published, the original studies have been repeated and extended with good results (Playfair personal communication). We have confirmed their observation in the NZB mice (18). Treatment of NZB mice at four weeks of age with syngeneic thymocytes from donors $\leq$ two weeks suppressed the direct Coombs test in all recipients (Figure 3) while the titer rose with age in controls (Figure 4). Spleen cells and bone marrow cells were not effective (Table VIII). Initiation of young thymocyte treatment at ten weeks of age rather than four weeks was ineffective (18).

DISCUSSION

Taken together, the studies described suggest that New Zealand mice lose suppressor function with age followed by the development of autoimmunity. Suppressor function appears to be lost at a time when helper function in intact. Whether this is due to shorter survival of suppressor cells, preferential premature decrease in production, an abnormality in maturation or some other process remains unknown.

It is possible that naturally occurring thymocytotoxic antibody (NTA) could be responsible for the loss of suppressor function by either direct or indirect effects (19)

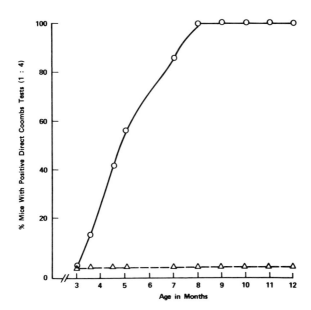

Figure 3. Four week old NZB mice were treated
with young thymocytes from syngeneic mice
(triangles) or medium (circles) and the cumu-
lative incidence of Coomb's positivity (a
titer of 1:4 or greater) recorded as the mice
aged.

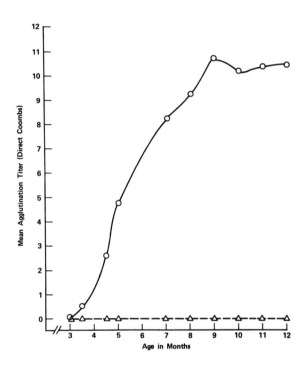

Figure 4. Direct Coomb's test titers of NZB
mice treated from four weeks of age with
syngeneic thymocytes from two week mice
(triangles) or medium alone (circles).

TABLE VIII

Suppression of anti-erythrocyte Antibodies
(measured by direct Coombs test)
in NZB Mice by Injections of Young
(≤ 2 weeks) Syngeneic Thymocytes Every Two Weeks

	Percentage of Mice Positive			
Treatment	Three months (%)	Five months (%)	Eight months (%)	Twelve months (%)
Medium only	0	55	100	100
Young thymocytes*	0	0	0	0
Young spleen cells*	0	43	100	ND[§]
Young marrow cells[†]	0	57	100	ND

*   *5 × 10^7 cells*

[†]   *3 × 10^6 cells*

[§]   *Not determined*

However, since NTA has been found to be of the IgM class, it
would not be expected to cross the placenta (19). It would,
therefore, be difficult to envisage its synthesis in
sufficient quantity to produce hyperresponsiveness to SRBC
in the first ten days of life (1) or even impaired tolerance
induction after three weeks of life (1). The latter
phenomenon seems closely related in time to the loss of
suppressor cells which occurs in NZB/W mice between three
and ten weeks of age. This is before significant titers of
NTA are present free in the serum in the hybrid. These

arguments do not rule out the possibility that NTA is active and bound to T cells before it is free in the serum; however, there is no evidence for such a phenomenon early in life (20). In fact, widespread T-cell coating might be expected to lead to an increase in lymphoid cells with surface immunoglobulin; instead, a reduction has been reported (21).

The presence of NTA is not strongly correlated with anti-nuclear antibody. In humans with SLE it has been associated with disease activity suggesting a secondary rather than a primary role (22). Nonetheless, it remains to be proved that NTA is the result rather than the cause of decreased suppressor cells.

The apparent premature loss of thymic regulatory function in New Zealand mice could be caused by any one of a number of other factors. Viruses have been implicated as etiologic agents in autoimmune diseases. It is possible that viral infection of the thymus could alter T-cell maturation and production. Viruses could additionally act as immune enhancers or transmit genetic information. It is possible that NZB mice are unique in their susceptibility or in their response to a common virus rather than that they are infected by an unusual one. Genetic factors predisposing to autoimmunity might be susceptibility to certain viruses as well as (or instead of) immunologic ones.

Despite the uncertainty surrounding the cause of the premature loss of suppressor function in New Zealand mice, it appears possible for replacement therapy to alter the development of autoimmunity. Such therapy has potential application for human autoimmune diseases such as SLE. However, one could not conveniently administer cells to patients with this syndrome. Perhaps a non-antigenic suppressor substance could be given. Even more desirable would be the restoration of immune regulatory function. Further study of normal regulatory processes will be necessary to better understand the basis for the abnormality in autoimmune states so that attempts at correction can be approached more intelligently.

REFERENCES

1. Talal, N. and Steinberg, A.D., *Current Topics in Microbiol. and Immunol., 64:* 79, 1974.

2. Baker, P.J., Stashak, P.W., Amsbaugh, D.F., Prescott, B. and Barth, R.F., J. Immunol., *105*: 1581, 1970.

3. Chused, T.M., Steinberg, A.D. and Parker, L.M., J. Immunol., *111*: 52, 1973.

4. Barthold, D.R., Kysela, S. and Steinberg, A.D., J. Immunol., *112*: 9, 1974.

5. Hardin, J.A., Chused, T.M. and Steinberg, A.D., J. Immunol., *111*: 650, 1973.

6. Gerber, N.L., Hardin, J.A., Chused, T.M. and Steinberg, A.D., J. Immunol., *113*: 1618, 1974.

7. Dutton, R.W., J. Exp. Med., *136*: 1445, 1972.

8. Rich, R.R. and Pierce, C.W., J. Exp. Med., *137*: 205, 1973.

9. Gershwin, M.E. and Steinberg, A.D., Proc. Soc. Exp. Biol. Med., *147*: 425, 1974.

10. Dauphinee, M.J. and Talal, N., Proc. Nat. Acad. Sci., *70*: 3769, 1973.

11. Gershon, R.K. and Kencin, R.S., J. Immunol., *107*: 359, 1971.

12. Bach, J.-F., Dardenne, M. and Salomon, J.-C., Clin. Exp. Immunol., *14*: 247, 1973.

13. Dauphinee, M.J., Talal, N., Goldstein, A.L. and White, A., Proc. Nat. Acad. Sci., *71*: 2637, 1974.

14. Gershwin, M.E., Ahmed, A., Steinberg, A.D., Thurman,G.B. and Goldstein, A.L., J. Immunol., *113:* 1068, 1974.

15. Steinberg, A.D., Law. L.W. and Talal, N., Arthritis Rheum., *13*: 369, 1970.

16. Kysela, S. and Steinberg, A.D., Clin. Immunol. Immunopathol., *2*: 133, 1973.

17. Allison, A.C., Denman, A.M. and Barnes, R.D., Lancet, *2*: 135, 1971.

18. Gershwin, M.E. and Steinberg, A.D., Clin. Immunol. Immunopathol., 1975, In Press.

19. Shirai, T. and Mellors, R.C., Proc. Nat. Acad. Sci., *68*: 1412, 1971.

20. Shirai, T., Yoshiki, T. and Mellors, R.C., Clin. Exp. Immunol., *12*: 455, 1972.

21. Stobo, J.D., Talal, N. and Paul, W.E., J. Immunol., *109*: 701, 1972.

22. Stastny, P. and Ziff, M., Clin. Exp. Immunol., *8*: 543, 1971.

DISCUSSION FOLLOWING PRESENTATION

by Dr. ALFRED D. STEINBERG

L. WASHINGTON: Is there a normal distribution of light
   chain subgroups in the NZB mice as compared with
   "normal" mice?

A. STEINBERG: I don't think that that's been studied with
   the care you would require. In general most of the
   immunoglobulin is kappa as is true of most mice, but
   I don't think that the question has been examined in
   detail.

R. GERSHON: There seem to be a couple of inconsistencies in
   your data. NZB mice make a lot of autoantibodies, but
   they don't generally seem to have delayed hypersensitivity reactions against "self" antigens. They are
   hard to make tolerant with respect to serum antibody,
   but readily rendered tolerant with respect to delayed
   hypersensitivity. You find at one age good suppressor
   activity in their thymocytes when you measure it in
   terms of GVH response, but not when you measure it in
   terms of the antibody response. This gets back to the
   idea that the reciprocal relationship between antibody
   titer and cellular immunity may be controlled by a
   T cell. Would your data fit the notion that you are
   getting good suppression of delayed hypersensitivity at
   a time when you are getting poor or absent suppression
   of antibody synthesis - i.e., at 8-12 weeks?

A. STEINBERG: The answer is no. We are not getting good
   suppression of delayed hypersensitivity after eight
   weeks of age. We are getting good antibody responses
   at that time. The idea that they behave in a reciprocal
   manner is correct, but suppressor cells both for
   delayed hypersensitivity and for antibody production
   are lost progressively between four and ten weeks. At

eight weeks suppressor activity is pretty well gone for
both delayed hypersensitivity and antibody production.

R. GERSHON: I saw in the data you presented that at eight
weeks you had good suppression of GVH. At eight weeks
Normal Talal says that the suppressor cells and the
ability to become tolerant are lacking in terms of the
HGG response and in terms of the DNA synthetic response
taking place in the spleen.

A. STEINBERG: One of the reasons why I started out dividing
the NZB from the NZB/W mice is that I think there is
significant variation in the ages at which the
different strains lose different subpopulations of cells.
Normal Talal has shown using Richard Gershon's system
(probably first demonstrated by Dr. Gershon himself)
that NZB mice at two weeks of age have a normal proliferative response in irradiated recipients (that is,
when their thymocytes are transferred to allogeneic
recipients). In contrast at eight weeks of age their
responsiveness in this system is abnormal. NZB mice in
our hands (and I believe this is a general phenomenon)
lose suppressor cells earlier than do NZB/NZW mice. So
it would not be inconsistent to find eight week old
mice in which the NZB/NZW mice still have some
suppressor activity.

G. THORBECKE: Can you further define the properties of the
suppressor thymocytes in the "Coombs test" suppression
study?

A. STEINBERG: I will have to tell you why these studies
were performed in order to answer that question
rationally. It was mentioned by Allison and coworkers
in an article in the Lancet several years ago that
Dr. Playfair had performed such experiments and
obtained a positive result. We have never seen the
actual data. However, we thought that we might be able
to suppress malignancy in the NZB mice by giving thymocytes. The studies were, therefore, set up primarily
to look at the suppression of lymphomas rather than at
the suppression of the Coombs test. As a result, we did
not ask the question that you are interested in. Those

studies are currently in progress, but I don't have any answers as yet. Thus, I do not yet know the detailed properties of the suppressor thymocytes.

I. SEIGEL: You showed in one experiment that suppressor activity is lost before helper activity. Do you have an explanation for this? Do you feel that this observation indicates that suppressor cells are different from helper cells?

A. STEINBERG: Our data don't really address that question. If one were to remove the thymus at four weeks of age, I think you would find that suppressor cells would be lost by seven weeks of age and that there would still be lots of helper cells around. Since suppressor cells seem to be more short-lived than helper cells, one would expect them to be lost faster. On the other hand, we do have some evidence which suggests that suppressors are different than helpers. Dr. Gershon feels strongly otherwise and I don't think that we have any data that are sufficiently inconsistent with this hypothesis to really make a strong case against it.

MECHANISMS OF IMMUNOLOGICAL TOLERANCE

David H. Katz

Department of Pathology,
Harvard Medical School, Boston, Massachusetts

INTRODUCTION

Immunological tolerance has stimulated the curiosity of immunologists for many years because, on the one hand, it is well understood that it is nature's provision to allow the complex mammalian organism to coexist within itself, and, on the other hand, although the phenomena of immunological tolerance have been well-defined, the cellular and molecular mechanisms underlying them remain largely enigmatic.

The recognition of the role of thymus-derived or T lymphocytes as regulatory cells for immune responses, endowed with the capacity to both facilitate and suppress the functions of other T lymphocytes and bone marrow-derived B lymphocytes in reactions of cell-mediated and humoral immunity, has clearly deepened our understanding of the control mechanisms involved in these responses. However, we are now faced with the increasing complexity that this understanding places on the concept of specific immunological tolerance. Accordingly, in recent years studies on the mechanisms of tolerance induction have focused upon the experimental conditions required to establish tolerance in one or the other of these classes of lymphocytes.

In this paper I will briefly summarize and review the current conceptual framework surrounding the mechanism(s) of specific immunological tolerance, as I view it, and I will reiterate some of our own previously published data to emphasize selected points in this framework.

ALTERNATIVE PATHWAYS TO SPECIFIC UNRESPONSIVENESS

There are essentially three major conceptual categories into which specific unresponsiveness can be divided--cell blockade, active suppression and clonal deletion (or abortion). These major categories are termed to reflect the predominant mechanistic consequence of one or more intervening events in a given pathway and, accordingly, each consists of perhaps several sub-categories. Moreover, as I will mention below, there is no *a priori* reason to consider these categories as absolutely distinct, since it is conceivable that unresponsiveness induced by mechanisms falling into one category (*i.e.* cell blockade)   may ultimately result in consequences of another category (*i.e.* clonal deletion). Upon this framework, one can formulate a broad descriptive summary of these major categories as follows.

I.   CELL BLOCKADE

The term "cell blockade" is poor and potentially misleading, but one is forced to use it in the absence of more precise knowledge of the mechanisms involved. What is meant by this term is the loss of reactivity of a population of specific immunocompetent lymphocytes as a direct consequence of interaction between antigenic determinants and the cell surface receptors binding such determinants under circumstances or conditions that are either particularly unfavorable to triggering or are particularly favorable to inactivation of the cells. In this category, which is clearly the broadest of the three, and probably the one most frequently interdigitating with the other two, fall in the following types of tolerance-inducing phenomena.

A.   *Antigen- Antibody Complexes*

The possible significance of antigen-antibody complexes in the induction of specific unresponsiveness has been indicated by the *in vitro* studies of Diener and Feldmann (reviewed in 1) in which an experimental model was designed to show that antigen-antibody complexes act as specific immunosuppressants at the level of the immunocompetent cell. This form of tolerance could be achieved with either immunogenic or subimmunogenic amounts of antigen complexed with antibody provided the complexes were formed within a critical ratio of antibody to antigen concentration

(excess of antigen). Although the initial experiments
suggested that such complexes induced tolerance in
specific B lymphocytes, subsequent studies have indicated
that antigen-antibody complexes are tolerogenic in
appropriate conditions for T cells as well (2). Into this
sub-category, I also place the phenomena ascribed to serum
"blocking" factors, since it has been suggested that such
factors consist of antigen-antibody complexes (3-5).

    B. *Determinant Concentration and Unique Molecular
Characteristics.*

        A number of studies have demonstrated the importance
of antigen dose to induction of tolerance *versus* immunity.
Perhaps the most familiar examples are the more frequently
used T-cell independent antigens such as pneumococcal polysaccharide (SIII) and polymerized flagellin (POL) which
display a very narrow dose range for immunity and above which
induce tolerance. The same has been found to be true of the
2,4-dinitrophenyl (DNP) derivatized copolymer of D-glutamic
acid and D-lysine (D-GL) which has been the subject of
extensive analysis in our laboratory (reviewed in 6 and 7).
Although most extensively studied for its potent tolerogenic
properties, DNP-D-GL has been recently shown to be immunogenic
in vitro at exceedingly low doses or when presented to
immunocompetent B cells as macrophage-bound molecules (8).
Thus, as is true of POL (9) or DNP-POL (10), the capacity of
DNP-D-GL and comparable molecules to induce immunity or
tolerance is a function of the determinant concentration
bound to the surface receptors of specific lymphocytes.
These differences can be obtained by either altering the dose
of antigen, or, in the case of haptenated derivatives, the
conjugation ratio of hapten per mole of carrier (10,11).

        There are certain molecules whose structural
properties lend to them rather unique properties insofar as
triggering immunity or tolerance. These are, in fact, the
very same class of T-independent antigens discussed above
and the structural features which they all share is a linear
sequence of repetitive units more or less equally spaced
along the molecule. This structural property appears to
allow binding of determinants in a suitable matrix for
induction of either immunity or tolerance depending on the
conditions at the cell surface such as epitope density. In
the case of at least two such molecules--i.e. DNP-D-GL and

POL--it has been shown that interaction of these determinants in appropriate concentrations with specific B cells prevents the normal sequence of receptor capping and endocytosis of antigen-receptor complexes (12,13), a point discussed further below.

C. *Antibody-mediated Unresponsiveness.*

In this sub-category, I am referring to specific inhibition of cell-mediated and humoral immune responses by reaction of cells with antisera containing antibodies directed against surface determinants of the lymphocytes. Noteworthy examples of this type of immunosuppression are: (a) the studies of Ramseier and Lindermann (14) and more recently by Wigzell and colleagues (15) demonstrating that antibodies raised against lymphocyte receptors specific for foreign alloantigens can effectively and specifically inhibit transplantation reactions--i.e. graft-versus-host; and (b) the studies reported by several investigators demonstrating inhibition of certain T cell and B cell responses with alloantisera directed against the histo-compatibility structures of the responding cells (16-18). Although I do not believe that such mechanisms are teleologically relevant, the great potential therapeutic importance of such experimental models demand their inclusion in any complete   list of mechanisms resulting in specific immunosuppression.

II. ACTIVE SUPPRESSION

This has become perhaps the most fashionable area of cellular immunology during the past two to three years as the pendulum of interest has swung away from the predominant attention paid to the positive or facilitating aspects of T-cell regulation of immune responses which originally appealed to most workers in the field. The subject has been reivewed extensively by its main proponents, notably Gershon (19) who, in fact, is contributing to this symposium, and therefore, I will devote only a moderate amount of space here to this topic. The main points that I wish to emphasize are that: (a) T-cell mediated suppression is an active process reflecting one end of the spectrum of T-cell regulatory influences on the immune system ranging from enhancement to suppression; (b) the suppressive

influences can be of a highly specific nature or of a totally nonspecific form; and (c) T-cell suppression can be
mediated on other T lymphocytes and on B lymphocytes.
These points will be illustrated in the experiment below.

    Perhaps the most revealing experiments in the studies
of cell-cell interactions have utilized systems in which
responses to hapten-carrier conjugates are assessed.
Although the enhancing effects of carrier-specific T cells
were recognized very early, the suppressive influences
exerted by such cells were not readily appreciated until
somewhat later. Among the first studies demonstrating this
dualistic influence of carrier-specific T cells in responses
to DNP-protein conjugates were those performed by us in
guinea pigs several years ago (20). A representative
experiment from these studies appears in Figure 1. The
guinea pigs in groups I-V were all primed with soluble DNP-
ovalbumin at week 0. One week later the various groups were
supplementally immunized in the footpads with a complete
Freund's adjuvant (CFA) emulsion containing 50 µg of either
bovine gamma globulin (BGG) or keyhole limpet hemocyanin
(KLH) or a mixture of BGG and KLH. Three weeks later
(week 4) guinea pigs were injected intraperitoneally (i.p.)
with 10 mg of either free soluble BGG or KLH or with saline.
One day thereafter all animals were secondarily challenged
with DNP-BGG. As summarized in Figure 1, the supplemental
immunization with BGG induces a population of BGG-specific
T cells capable of regulating the response to DNP-BGG. The
net effect is usually one of enhancement, under the
conditions employed, resulting in a very strong secondary
anti-DNP response to DNP-BGG (group I). {Although not
shown, it should be remembered that in the absence of BGG
supplemental immunization, DNP-OVA-primed animals would be
unable to mount secondary anti-DNP responses to DNP-BGG}.
However, administration of soluble unconjugated BGG one day
prior to secondary challenge virtually abrogates the
secondary response to DNP-BGG (group II). This remarkable
suppressive effect is clearly BGG-specific since
administration of unconjugated KLH to guinea pigs
supplementally immunized with only BGG in CFA fails to
appreciably suppress the response (group III).

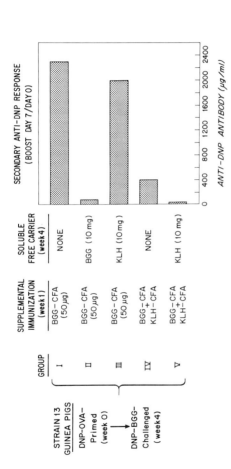

Figure 1. Specific and non-specific suppression of anti-hapten antibody responses in guinea pigs by administration of free carrier or by simultaneous supplemental immunization with two unrelated carriers.

Another form of suppression is illustrated by the results obtained in group IV. These guinea pigs developed markedly lower secondary anti-DNP antibody responses to DNP-BGG in comparison to group I as a consequence of having been supplementally (and simultaneously) immunized with both BGG and KLH. This effect must be considered to be non-antigen-specific since the final challenge involves DNP-BGG. Moreover, the administration of free soluble KLH one day prior to secondary challenge further increases the degree of suppression, provided KLH had been administered as a supplemental immunization (cf. group V with group III).

These results illustrate in one experiment the two types of T-cell-mediated suppression--i.e. specific and non-specific--which now have been documented by many independent investigators (19). To avoid becoming somewhat misleading in this regard, I shall define here the differences, as I view them, between the phenomena of specific and non-specific suppression.

A. *Specific Suppression.*

Specific suppression is that form which is perhaps most frequently involved in physiologic immune responses and consists of suppression of specific T cells with the same (or highly cross-reactive) determinant specificity. The net effect of this T-T cell interaction in humoral responses is to diminish the activity of helper T cells which in turn diminishes the response of the B cells being helped by such cells. This is illustrated by groups I-III in Figure 1 and has also been shown in similar *in vivo* systems by Basten (2) and by Tada (22) and appears to be analogous in mechanism to the specific suppression of cell-mediated immunity described by Zembala and Asherson (23) and Claman et al. (24). It is also likely that specific suppression can be exerted by T cells directly on B cells of the same specificity. An example of this is found in the studies of Kapp et al. (25) in the immune response (*Ir*) gene-controlled responses to the terpolymer glutamic acid-alanine-tyrosine (GAT) in mice. In this system mice lacking the relevant *Ir* gene fail to develop GAT-specific antibody responses under normal conditions but can be shown to produce GAT-specific suppressor T cells following administration of appropriate doses of GAT. These suppressor cells can then be shown to specifically suppress anti-GAT responses of spleen cells

from other mice that have been exposed to GAT complexed with
an immunogenic carrier under conditions that would otherwise
elicit GAT antibody responses (25). Another example of T-
cell suppression of B-cell function that may, however, be of
different specificity is the allotype suppression system in
mice that has been studied extensively by Herzenberg and
coworkers (reviewed in 26). An intriguing and perhaps
analogous phenomenon has been recently described by Waldmann
et al. (27) in certain hypogammaglobulinemic human patients
who appear to have aberrant suppressor T cells which act to
inhibit immunoglobulin synthesis and/or secretion by
B lymphocytes.

B. *Non-specific Suppression.*

Non-specific suppression is that which is a general
effect not necessarily related to a particular specificity
of response. This is shown by groups IV and V of Figure 1
in which KLH immunization suppresses the activity of DNP-
specific B cells and/or BGG-specific T cells. It is not
possible usually to determine the target cell of such
suppression or "antigenic competition" particularly in
responses to T-dependent antigens since either T cells, B
cells or macrophages (or combinations) could be suitable for
targets. This type of effect can be elicited by non-
specific T-cell mitogens and by T-dependent antigens but not
by T-independent antigens, thereby indicating the necessary
participation of T cells in the reactions. It is probable
that these non-specific suppressive effects reflect the
release of quantities of non-specific mediators that create
an uncomfortable milieu in the lymphoid tissue microenvironment.

III. CLONAL DELETION AND ABORTION

The deletion of specific clones of self-reactive
lymphocytes constitutes a central point in the clonal
selection theory proposed by Burnet (28). As originally
conceived, this notion assumed that potentially self-reactive
lymphocytes would encounter self antigens at very early
stages of differentiation at a time when the only inductive
stimulus capable of being received by such cells was a
tolerogenic or paralyzable signal (28,29). Recently, Nossal
and Pike (30) have refined the terminology to "clone

abortion" to distinguish this possible mechanism from
clonal deletion which implies the removal of fully competent
lymphocytes. Moreover, Nossal has correctly pointed out that
the concept has become recently unpopular in view of the
great facility with which fully mature and immunocompetent
lymphocytes can be rendered unresponsive in appropriate
experimental models. However, it is now clear that multiple
mechanistic pathways exist resulting in specific tolerance
and one or more of these pathways may ultimately lead to
deletion of the specific lymphocyte clone involved.

There is documented evidence in systems of B-cell
tolerance, where the specific lymphocytes are more readily
quantitated, that antigen-binding B cells are substantially
diminished in such conditions. This has been shown in the
DNP-D-GL tolerance system (31) and in the tolerance induced
by deaggregated human gamma globulin (32). It is pertinent
to note here that in both of these systems the state of
B-cell tolerance is irreversible once induced and presumably
requires regeneration of new cells from the stem cell pool
before responsiveness is once again established. There is no
direct evidence as to the fate of such tolerant cells,
however, demanding that we consider clonal deletion in the
functional rather than the absolute sense in these circumstances. The validity of the clonal abortion concept--i.e.
the elimination of specific clones of lymphocytes as a
result of antigen encounter at early maturation stages--has
been strengthened by very recent studies of Nossal and his
colleagues (30) but considerably more experimental documen-
tation of this type will probably be necessary to place this
issue in unequivocal terms.

QUALIFICATIONS AND INTERRELATIONSHIPS
AMONG THE ALTERNATIVE PATHWAYS TO UNRESPONSIVENESS

The three categories described above take into account
several pathways to an end result of functional unresponsiveness of immunocompetent lymphocytes but do not provide any
insight on the mechanisms involved at the cellular or
molecular level. Indeed, at the present time, we are not
very enlightened about the nature of such molecular events.

However, we do know certain facts that allow some tentative
conclusions or predictions to be made.

First, it is clear that the presence or absence of T-
cell participation at a critical time related to the binding
of antigen by specific B cells plays a major role in determining whether or not the inductive stimulus to the B cell
will be immunogenic or tolerogenic. This is dramatically
illustrated by studies in the DNP-D-GL tolerance system in
which the induction of a potent, non-specific, T-cell stimulus provided by a transient graft-*versus*-host reaction
(allogeneic effect) converts a normally tolerogenic signal
into an immunogenic one (reviewed in 33). It is important,
however, that such T-cell participation occurs either before
or concomitant with the exposure to the tolerogen since
once the tolerogenic signal has been received, the B cells
are not susceptible to reversal or "rescue". Similar
conditions have been discussed at length by Mitchell
concerning the relative ease of B-cell tolerance induction by
T-dependent antigens in mice relatively deficient in T cells
such as is the case of congenitally athymic nude mice (34).

Secondly, there appear to be two functionally distinct
phases of unresponsiveness, namely, reversible and
irreversible, and the difference between them depends on
multiple determining factors such as time, antigen dose,
molecular properties, etc. The important point of distinc-
tion is that one form of unresponsiveness is subject to
reversal by various means for at least a finite period of
time. Thus, the specific cell binding antigen of a common
molecular structure in free solution and under conditions of
moderate epitope density in the absence of T-cell participation can probably undergo three alternative pathways:
(a) The cell, because of avidity considerations among other
things, may shed the antigen very rapidly even before
significant amounts are interiorized and remain normally
responsive. This possibility is of trivial interest to
considerations of tolerance mechanisms and is pointed out
only for completeness of the alternatives. (b) The cell
having completed the sequence of antigen binding with
subsequent capping, interiorization and receptor resynthesis
might encounter helper T-cell activity of either a specific
or non-specific nature induced within a critical time period
after the B-cell binding events have occurred. The element
of time here seems to be of utmost and determining importance

to either prevent or result in the final alternative. (c) In
the absence of T-cell helper activity for a finite period
time, the B cell having undergone the first stages of cell-
antigen interaction now realizes it is lost and slips into a
state of irreversible tolerance.

The critical time during which a B cell is reversibly
refractory most logically differs depending upon conditions
of antigen concentration, etc. but has the common feature
of inevitably resulting in irreversible tolerance if no
appropriate intervention occurs. Precisely what intervention
is appropriate is obscure but it is intriguing to consider
that one of the important aspects of reversal is related to
the effects on certain critical cell surface sites (other
than immunoglobulin receptors) that might be the same or
similar to the surface molecules involved in physiologic T-B-
cell interactions.

The latter sequence is one more probably involved in
physiologic mechanisms of tolerance. It is quite conceivable
for example, that B cells with specific receptors for auto-
antigens that may be constantly originating from the stem
cell pool are rendered tolerant in this manner by virtue of
undergoing the antigen-binding sequence in absence of T-cell
helper functions. Likewise, the development of autoantibody
production is understandable when conditions allowing for
non-specific or cross-reactive T-cell activation arise as,
for example, with chronic infections.

Finally, although the aforementioned sequence alludes to
the consequence of antigen binding in the <u>absence</u> of T cell
participation, it is not unlikely that the consequences of
suppressor T-cell functions are precisely the same, and
perhaps for the same reasons--i.e. <u>absence</u> of helper T-cell
function. This reasoning is stimulated by the point
emphasized above that <u>suppressor</u> T cells, at least of the
antigen-specific variety, might well act to a major degree by
suppressing <u>helper</u> T cells of the same specificity. Since
the obvious net effect of this balance should in some circumstances be the cancelling out of helper function, the B cell
would, therefore, be in the predicament of becoming
irreversibly tolerant. To what extent suppressor activity
of T cells or macrophages may directly affect B cells, and if
so, by what cellular mechanisms must await more detailed

analysis.

MECHANISMS OF TOLERANCE INDUCTION
IN EITHER T OR B LYMPHOCYTES

In the preceding sections, I have emphasized the categories of pathways resulting in tolerance in terms of the
general conditions determining such pathways, such as antigen
dose, timing, etc. In this section I will focus on the
mechanisms described above as they pertain to each of the two
lymphocyte classes. In essence, this will necessarily
result in some repetition of the points made previously but
now placed in the context of the B or T lymphocytes.

The available data indicate that B lymphocytes are
rendered unresponsive by mechanisms in all three categories.
Indeed, cell blockade by antigen-antibody complexes and by
determinant concentration and/or molecular structural
properties of antigens binding to specific B cells have been
demonstrated most often in responses of this lymphocyte class.
The cell blockade phenomena resulting from exposure to alloantisera or anti-alloantibodies have not clearly been shown
to induce unresponsiveness in B lymphocytes so this possible
mechanism remains open. The induction of unresponsiveness in
B cells as a consequence of suppressor T-cell function is
probably reflected in the *Ir* gene-controlled GAT system in
mice, the allotype suppression phenomenon and the cases of
hypogammaglobulinemia described above. It is not as yet
defined, however, whether such unresponsiveness in B cells is
a direct consequence of suppressor T cells (or their products)
acting on such cells, or rather, an indirect consequence
resulting from inadequate helper T-cell function due to
direct suppression of the latter cell type. Clonal deletion
has been observed in experimental models of B-cell tolerance
where it has been possible to detect and quantitate specific
antigen-binding B-cell precursors. The manner in which such
B cells are lost is still an open question, however, since
the cells may either be lost by phagocytosis and cell death
or alternatively, remain viable but in an afunctional state
with no capacity for synthesis and/or expression of cell
surface receptors.

The mechanisms involved in T-cell tolerance are not as clearly defined as is the case with B lymphocytes. Cell blockade phenomena appear to inactivate T cells in certain instances--i.e. antigen-antibody complexes and alloantisera-- but not in others. For example, whereas hapten-D-GL conjugates are highly tolerogenic for B cells, these same molecules fail to induce T-cell tolerance (35,36). Whether this difference reflects distinct binding characteristics or crucial differences in molecular pathways of activation and inactivation between these two lymphocyte classes remains to be determined. Active suppression has been shown to be an important mechanisms of T-cell inactivation in cell-mediated immunity (19,23,24) as well as cooperative T-cell functions (20-22). Functional clone deletion has been shown to occur in T-cell populations in models of tolerance induction to protein antigens in conditions where no suppressor T-cell activity appears to exist (32). As is the case with B lymphocytes, however, it is not known whether functional deletion of T cells is equivalent to cell death or not.

CONCLUSIONS

The studies presented here serve to focus not only on two distinctive forms of B-cell tolerance but also on certain of the fundamental issues to which investigations on the phenomenology of tolerance should be primarily directed, namely, potential applicability of the model systems employed to clinical use and relevance of what is learned to mechanisms of self tolerance.

The potential clinical applicability of tolerance systems such as that represented by DNP-D-GL could be enormous. The properties of the D-GL molecule and presumably other structurally similar substances that promote inactivation of specific B lymphocytes binding determinants attached to D-GL opens a wide area of deleterious antibody production to attack. Since studies thus far have delineated the potent tolerogenic properties of D-GL bearing small, well defined determinants, the immediate practical possibilities include tolerization in patients with hypersensitivity to the

benzylpenicilloyl determinants of penicillin and its
analogues. More dramatic application would be the use of
D-GL bearing nucleotide and nucleoside determinants to
abolish anti-nuclear antibody production in patients with
systemic lupus erythematosus (SLE). Indeed, recent studies
in our laboratory have demonstrated that nucleoside-D-GL
complexes can effectively abrogate anti-nuclear antibody
production in mice (37) and long-term investigations of the
effects of these molecules in the pathogenesis of autoimmune
disease in NZB mice are currently being undertaken. In
another area of perhaps the largest potential usefulness,
namely, treatment of common immediate hypersensitivity
disease states, the groundwork is being laid but a vast
amount of further research is essential. Thus, we have
established the fact that determinants coupled to D-GL will
effectively tolerize B cells of the IgE class as well as
other antibody classes (38). However, what is not yet
determined is whether more complex multi-determinant antigens
will be tolerogenic to B cells once coupled to D-GL. This
will be absolutely necessary if one is to consider the
possible induction of tolerance in patients with hay fever by
administering purified ragweed antigens coupled to D-GL.
Studies currently underway in our laboratory should resolve
this issue in one way or another in the not too distant
future. Finally, of course, if any of these possible
therapeutic applications are to be achieved, it will be
essential to determine methods by which these substances can
be administered to the patient with relative impunity to his
or her health.

The issue of relevance of the various experimental
models of B-cell tolerance to the mechanisms of self-
tolerance remains highly conjectural, but a reasonably
educated framework of thought can be derived from the available systems being studied. If the assumption is made that
T cells specific for self-antigens capable of providing helper
function for B cells do not exist {for reasons considered in
greater depth elsewhere (39)}, then the functional inactivation of B cells specific for auto-antigens may occur via the
following pathway primarily in relation to the concentrations
of the self-antigens concerned. Thus, in the case of self-
antigens in high concentrations and ready accessibility--
i.e. serum proteins, circulating histocompatibility antigen
molecules, etc.--specific B cells arising from the stem cell
pool become virtually bathed in these antigens and are
routinely inactivated perhaps even very early in their

differentiation pathway. Cells possessing specific receptors
for binding these self-antigens would not, therefore, be
expected to be detected at least by the currently available
techniques. On the other hand, in the case of self-antigens
that exist in relatively low quantities sequestered perhaps
in selected tissue sites--i.e. thyroglobulin--,it would be
understandable why B cells specific for such antigens might
be rather easily found, as indeed they have in recent years.
The presumption follows, however, that the B cells detected
have not themselves been exposed to an appreciable extent to
the antigen--those which have contacted the antigen in
sufficient amounts and for a sufficient duration of time are
either inactivated or in the process of becoming so,
provided helper T-cell activity is lacking. In the event
that some form of (e.g. non-specific) T-cell help occurs--
for example, during a chronic infectious process involving
release of significant quantities of adjuvant substances--
then autoantibody production may readily ensue and be of
either transient or more prolonged duration depending on the
circumstances.

    How then does the inactivation sequence occur in such
B cells following the binding of self-antigens in the
absence of helper T-cell function. If, as appears to be the
case, B cells can bind, cap, interiorize or catabolize the
antigen molecules and resynthesize their surface receptors
in the absence of helper T cells (40), then it is possible
to envisage that either after one or perhaps after several
such cycles of antigen-binding receptor resynthesis the cell
may be induced to undergo terminal blast transformation, thus,
eliminating it from the available cell pool. The absence of
a helper T-cell influence, therefore, results in a normal
pathway to this end result (terminal blastogenesis) with no
capability for further differentiation into antibody-
producing or memory cells (clonal deletion). If the
evidence becomes clear that suppressor T cells may be
involved in the maintenance of some forms of self-tolerance
and that such involvement is a direct effect on B lymphocytes
then the possibility must be considered that such suppressor
T cells accomplish their functional effects likewise by
stimulating B cells to undergo terminal differentiation.
Definitive answers to these possibilities may be soon forth-
coming.

ACKNOWLEDGMENTS

I am grateful to all of my colleagues who participated in the studies from our laboratory discussed herein, in particular to Professor Baruj Benacerraf for critical review of the manuscript.

I am also grateful to Miss Deborah Maher for secretarial assistance.

This work was supported by Grant AI-10630 from the National Institutes of Health.

REFERENCES

1. Diener, E. and Feldmann, M., Transplant. Rev., 8: 76, 1972.

2. Feldmann, M. and Nossal, G.J.V., Transplant. Rev., 13: 3, 1972.

3. Sjögren, H.O., Hellström, I., Barsal, S.C. and Hellström, K.E., Proc. Nat. Acad. Sci. (U.S.), 68: 1372, 1971.

4. Wright, P.W., Hargreaves, R.E., Barsal, S.C., Bernstein, I.D. and Hellström, K.E., Proc. Nat. Acad. Sci. (U.S.), 70: 2539, 1973.

5. Baldwin, R.W., Price, M.R. and Robius, R.A., Int. J. Cancer, 11: 527, 1973.

6. Katz, D.H., in *Immunological Tolerance: Mechanisms and Potential Therapeutic Applications,* Edited by D.H. Katz and B. Benacerraf, p. 189, Academic Press, New York, 1974.

7. Katz, D.H. and Benacerraf, B., in *Immunological Tolerance: Mechanisms and Potential Therapeutic Applications*, Edited by D.H. Katz and B. Benacerraf, p. 249, Academic Press, New York, 1974.

8. Paul, W.E., Karpf, M. and Mosier, D.E., in *Immunological Tolerance: Mechanisms and Potential Therapeutic Applications*, Edited by D.H. Katz and B. Benacerraf, p. 141, Academic Press, New York, 1974.

9. Diener, E. and Armstrong, W.D., J. Exp. Med., *129*: 591, 1969.

10. Feldmann, M., J. Exp. Med., *135*: 735, 1972.

11. Desaymard, C., Feldmann, M. and Maurer, P., in *Immunological Tolerance: Mechanisms and Potential Therapeutic Applications*, Edited by D.H. Katz and B. Benacerraf, p. 225, Academic Press, New York, 1974.

12. Diener, E., in *Immunological Tolerance: Mechanisms and Potential Therapeutic Applications*, Edited by D.H. Katz and B. Benacerraf, p. 543, Academic Press, New York, 1974.

13. Ault, K.A., Unanue, E.R., Katz, D.H. and Benacerraf, B., Proc. Nat. Acad. Sci. (U.S.), *71*: 3111, 1974.

14. Ramseier, H. and Lindenmann, J., Transplant. Rev., *10*: 57, 1972.

15. Binz, H., Lindenmann, J. and Wigzell, H., J. Exp. Med., *140*: 731, 1974.

16. Shevach, E.M., Paul, W.E. and Green, I., J. Exp. Med., *136*: 1207, 1972.

17. Shevach, E.M., Green, I. and Paul, W.E., J. Exp. Med., *139*: 679, 1974.

18. Pierce, C.W., Kapp, J.A., Solliday, S.M., Dorf, M.E. and Benacerraf, B., J. Exp. Med., *140*: 921, 1974.

19. Gershon, R.K., Contemp. Topics Immunobiol., *3*: 1, 1974.

20. Katz, D.H., Paul, W.E. and Benacerraf, B., J. Immunol., *110*: 107, 1972.

21. Basten, A., in *Immunological Tolerance: Mechanisms and Potential Therapeutic Applications*, Edited by D.H. Katz and B. Benacerraf, p. 107, Academic Press, New York, 1974.

22. Tada, T., in *Immunological Tolerance: Mechanisms and Potential Therapeutic Applications*, Edited by D.H. Katz and B. Benacerraf, p. 471, Academic Press, New York, 1974.

23. Zembala, M. and Asherson, G.L., Nature, *244*: 227, 1973.

24. Claman, H.N., Phanuphak, P. and Moorhead, J.W., in *Immunological Tolerance: Mechanisms and Potential Therapeutic Applications*, Edited by D.H. Katz and B. Benacerraf, p. 123, Academic Press, New York, 1974.

25. Kapp, J.A., Pierce, C.W., Schlossman, S. and Benacerraf, B., J. Exp. Med., *140*: 648, 1974.

26. Herzenberg, L.A. and Herzenberg, L.A., Contemp. Topics Immunobiol., *3*: 41, 1974.

27. Waldmann, T.A., Broder, S., Blaese, R.M., Durm, M., Blackman, M. and Strober, W., Lancet, *2*: 609, 1974.

28. Burnet, F.M., *The Clonal Selection Theory of Acquired Immunity*, Cambridge University Press, 1959.

29. Lederberg, J., Science, *129*: 1649, 1959.

30. Nossal, G.J.V. and Pike, B.L., in *Immunological Tolerance: Mechanisms and Potential Therapeutic Applications*, Edited by D.H. Katz and B. Benacerraf, p. 351, Academic Press, New York, 1974.

31. Katz, D.H., Davie, J.M., Paul, W.E. and Benacerraf, B., J. Exp. Med., *134*: 201, 1971.

32. Louis, J.A., Chiller, J.M. and Weigle, W.O., J. Exp. Med., *138*: 1481, 1973.

33. Katz, D.H., Transplant. Rev., *12*: 141, 1972.

34. Mitchell, G.F., in *Immunological Tolerance: Mechanisms and Potential Therapeutic Applications*, Edited by D.H. Katz and B. Benacerraf, p. 283, Academic Press, New York, 1974.

35. Benacerraf, B. and Katz, D.H., J. Immunol., *112*: 1158, 1974.

36. Bullock, W.W., Katz, D.H. and Benacerraf, B., J. Immunol., 1975, in press.

37. Eshhar, Z., Benacerraf, B. and Katz, D.H., J. Immunol., *114*: 000, 1975.

38. Katz, D.H., Hamaoka, T. and Benacerraf, B., Proc. Nat. Acad. Sci. (U.S.), *70*: 2776, 1973.

39. Katz, D.H. and Benacerraf, B., Transplant. Rev., *22*: 000, 1975.

40. Ault, K.A. and Unanue, E.R., J. Exp. Med., *139*: 1110, 1974.

DISCUSSION FOLLOWING PRESENTATION

by DR. DAVID H. KATZ

R. GERSHON: First I would like to complement you on the
    manner in which you covered the entire field of
    tolerance so clearly. Then I would like to take issue
    with the point you make that mature B cells presented
    with antigen in the absence of T-cell help become
    tolerant. The only evidence that this occurs is in
    your system with DNP-GL. It has not been demonstrated
    with any other antigen.

D. KATZ: I really must disagree with you in that regard.
    Several other workers including John Schrader and
    John Hamilton have arrived at conclusions similar to
    ours based upon studies in completely different systems.
    In addition, there is the work of Graham Mitchell and
    others which is consistent with the findings we have
    reported.

R. GERSHON: We really don't have time to discuss all of
    these systems in detail. I would like to raise one
    other question. Regarding your category of "blockade",
    recent evidence has suggested that suppression mechanisms
    may be involved in several of the models you have placed
    in the "blockade" classification. In particular, it has
    been shown that antigen-antibody complexes do activate
    suppressor T cells. Also recent work by Gelfand and
    Paul has raised interesting questions regarding the
    mechanism of the action of anti-allosera. Mice treated
    with anti-theta antisera develop large populations of
    suppressor T cells which when transferred to other
    animals suppress their immune response.

R. SHANDAR: I was delighted with your presentation of the
    basic concepts of immunological tolerance. What is
    your feeling about the relationship of tolerance to

immunotherapy of tumors in which patients may be receiving multiple injections of cells? In some centers they are giving 10^9 or 10^{10} allogeneic myeloblasts. How do you view the T- B-cell interaction in relation to the varying doses of these cells? Do you think it is possible that these patients develop tolerance by such procedures to tissue antigens or to leukemia associated antigens?

D. KATZ: I really don't know a good answer to give you. It is a situation where experience will be the main teacher. I would personally doubt that such procedures would lead to tolerance. Of course, many of these patients are immunosuppressed to begin with or on immunosuppressive drugs. This does raise some additional problems for prediction. I don't think that there is any good experimental evidence which can provide an answer to your question.

I. SEIGEL: I would like to ask you to comment on the concept of tolerance susceptible periods, such as after irradiation.

D. KATZ: It has been shown by several investigators that at very early ages animals are loaded with T cells that are readily made into suppressor T cells. After irradiation I would presume the same situation exists becuase it is my own personal bias to believe that suppressor T cells represent an earlier stage in the ultimate differentiation pathway of T lymphocytes. Thus, I would expect that during regeneration after x-irradiation there would be a relative abundance of suppressor T cells as compared with helper T cells.

DISCUSSION by DR. HANS WIGZELL

I would like to talk about evidence for "suppressor" B cells suppressing specific T cells. Let us let A and C stand for the major histocompatibility loci antigens in in-bred rats. The assumption is that one can talk about antibodies without distinguishing between T and B-cell anti-bodies. Then an AA animal has the capacity to make A anti-C, but lacks the capacity to make anti-A. Idiotypic antibodies against self-antigens are absent in the animal. You can show that inoculation of AA T cells or A anti-C alloantibodies stimulates the production, in an F_1 hybrid, of antibody that carries the reactivity anti-(A anti-C). The F_1 hybrid can make both IgM and IgG anti-idiotype antibodies. Most likely this is a T-dependent response. We can show that such anti-bodies are clearly idiotypic. If you now make A anti-C or A anti-B antibodies you can demonstrate in Ouchterlony plates a line of precipitation between the anti-(A anti-C) and the A anti-C but not with the A anti-B. This establishes the idiotypic specificity of the anti-(A anti-C) antibody made in the F_1 animal. This is very similar to the work of Fitch and his colleagues in Chicago. They actually found such an anti-idiotype antibody formed in hyperimmunized animals as an autoantibody response. It is possible that when one forms circulating immune complexes the antigen in the complex can stimulate helper T cells permitting B cells to make anti-idiotypic autoantibodies.

A striking experiment which we have done recently is as follows: If you immunize an F_1 (A x C) with purified A strain T cells then the F_1 hybrid can make anti-(A anti-C) which can react either with IgG antibodies produced in AA animals or with purified normal A strain T cells. In fact as far as we can see with our data the T and the B lymphocytes of AA animals which react with C antigens share idiotypic determinants. The important part of this is that such an immunized F_1 hybrid can be shown to be resistant to the graft-vs-host (GVH) reaction of AA cells. An F_1 hybrid can be shown to be resistant to the graft-vs-host (GVH) reaction of AA cells. An F_1 hybrid is generally thought of as being incapable of reacting against parental strain antigens. In

fact, however, it is capable of reacting against idiotypic
determinants present on the AA cells. Normal AA cells
treated with this anti-idiotype antiserum, in the presence of
complement, are completely inactivated with respect to their
ability to react with C either in the GVH reaction or in
mixed lymphocyte culture while they retain their normal
capacity to react against another alloantigen, say E. Thus,
we can show that we have an anti-idiotypic antiserum which
can specifically eliminate those cells bearing the anti-C
idiotype. In fact, we can now actually determine the percentage, in normal animals, of A anti-C B cells and T cells.

    We can never detect any anti-self idiotype positive
lymphocytes. Here is an example of a "suppressor" B cell.
The anti-idiotype antibody is of course a B-cell product.
This product of B cells (anti-idiotype antibody) has the
capacity to selectively inactivate B or T cells carrying the
relevant idiotype. It is possible in diseases where you have
antigen-antibody complexes present that such an anti-
idiotype antibody can be produced and can not only selectively wipe out the B-cell capacity to react, but also
selectively eliminate the T-cell capacity to react.

QUESTIONS FOLLOWING DISCUSSION

by DR. HANS WIGZELL

J. HAMILTON: Is it possible that the apparent idiotypic
determinant on the T cell is really cytophilic antibody?

H. WIGZELL: I think not. First if you look at the distribution of the density of idiotype positive receptors
(on normal cells, not immune cells) you find a highly
discontinuous pattern. The majority are non-labelled
and a few are highly labelled (using autoradiography or
fluorescence techniques). The density of antigen-
binding receptors on T lymphocytes is very similar to
that of B cells in our hands. Secondly, if you remove
the idiotype positive receptors by proteolytic enzyme
treatment of purified T cells then the cells regain the
idiotype receptor upon culture. The molecule that they
make is not the same as that made by B-cell although
the idiotype is the same.

G.J. THORBECKE: Is the frequency of reactive cells high?

H. WIGZELL: The idiotype bearing cells are polyclonal.

MECHANISM OF ANTIBODY MEDIATED IMMUNE SUPPRESSION

Gregory W. Siskind

*Division of Allergy and Immunology, Department of Medicine
Cornell University Medical College, New York, New York*

It has been known for many years that passive antibody injected simultaneously with or soon after antigen can specifically depress antibody synthesis. The suppression of antibody synthesis by passive antibody was first reported in 1909 by Smith (1). This phenomenon has been extensively studied since then and the literature dealing with it has been reviewed by Uhr and Möller (2). In general, suppression is highly specific. The degree of suppression is directly related to the dose of passive antibody administered and inversely related to the amount of antigen used for immunization. The greater the time interval between immunization and subsequent injection of passive antibody, the less effective is the passive antibody in suppressing antibody synthesis. Usually it is easier to suppress the primary antibody response than to suppress priming to give a secondary response or to suppress a secondary response. Suppression can be produced with Fab or Fab_2 fragments but perhaps with somewhat reduced efficiency as compared with intact antibody. Passive antibody has also been shown to be capable of inhibiting both sensitization to give a delayed hypersensitivity reaction and the expression of delayed hypersensitivity by a sensitized animal.

Elegant experiments by Uhr and co-workers (3,4) established that suppression operated *in vivo* as a mechanism to control the magnitude of the immune response. In essence, these workers succeeded in acutely reducing the serum concentration of a specific antibody in an immunized animal by use of exchange transfusion or immunoadsorbents. The animals promptly began to synthesize increased amounts of the antibody that was specifically depleted so that its serum concentration rapidly exceeded that expected at the time in

immunization at which the studies were performed. Other
antibodies showed no change in concentration as a result of
the manipulation establishing the specificity of this control
mechanism.

Recently the phenomenon of antibody mediated immune
suppression has been adopted for clinical use (5). It has
been established that passive antibody to Rh positive cells
will specifically suppress the immune response of humans to
these antigens. The injection of such antiserum is now used
routinely to prevent the development of anti-Rh antibodies
in Rh negative mothers giving birth to Rh positive offspring
thus protecting against development of *erythroblastosis
fetalis* in future pregnancies. Details of this pharmacologi-
cal use of immune suppression will be presented in another
paper at this symposium (6).

It is generally believed that the mechanism of antibody
mediated immune suppression is the binding of antigen by
serum antibody thus blocking the interaction of antigen with
potential antibody-forming cells. In this manner, antibody
would block the selection and stimulation of potential antibody-forming cells. Presumably antibody could block interaction of antigen with both T and B cells. The properties of
antibody mediated suppression described above are all consistent with this hypothesis for the mechanism of suppression.
For example, the fact that it is more difficult to suppress a
secondary response or priming as compared with primary antibody synthesis is consistent with observations indicating
that in general elicitation of a secondary response or
priming can be accomplished with a lower dose of antigen than
is required to elicit primary antibody synthesis. The fact
that Fab or Fab_2 fragments can suppress is consistent with
binding of antigen as the critical feature of suppression. I
would like to consider, in this paper, the effect of suppression on several other aspects of the immune response in particular the affinity of the antibody formed. I would also
like to describe several additional experimental tests of the
hypothesis offered above to explain suppression.

Before proceeding to presentation of data, I would like
to discuss briefly the theoretical basis for studies on
heterogeneity of antibody affinity. By affinity is meant the
strength of the chemical bond formed between the antigenic

determinant and the antibody combining site. This property
of the reaction of antigen and antibody is expressed either
as the association constant (equilibrium constant, K) for the
reaction of antibody with a univalent ligand (hapten) or as
the free energy change (ΔF^O) occurring in that reaction as
calculated from the association constant by the usual
relationships. For the reaction of an antibody combining
site (Ab) with univalent hapten (H) one can write:

$$Ab + H \rightleftarrows AbH$$

$$K = \frac{(AbH)}{(Ab)(H)}$$

$$\Delta F^O = -RT \ln K$$

In these equations:

K = association constant.

Ab,H,AbH = the molar concentration of antibody, hapten and
antibody-hapten complexes respectively at
equilibrium.

ΔF^O = free energy change for the reaction (a more
negative free energy change indicating a higher
affinity antibody).

R = gas constant.

T = absolute temperature for the reaction.

ln K = natural logarithm of the association constant.

It is well known that the antibody formed by an
individual animal is highly heterogeneous with respect to its
affinity for the antigenic determinant (7,8). In addition

it has been shown that the "average" affinity of the
population of antibody molecules increases progressively
with time after immunization (8-10). The rate of increase
in affinity is faster with lower doses of antigen (8-10).
These observations have been interpreted (11,12) in terms of
a clonal selection hypothesis such as originally proposed by
Burnet (13). According to such a theory, B lymphocytes have
on their surface antibody molecules with antigen binding
properties identical to those of the antibody which that cell
and its progeny, will secrete after stimulation by antigen.
This "cell associated" antibody serves to capture antigen.
The interaction of antigen (perhaps after some preliminary
processing, localization or interaction with T cells and/or
macrophages) with cell associated antibody on B lymphocytes
selects that cell to proliferate and secrete antibody.
This selection process operates in addition to any other
possible mechanism which may be required to trigger B-cell
proliferation. Clearly B cells bearing high affinity cell
associated antibody will have an advantage in capturing and
retaining antigen especially at low antigen concentrations.
In this way, high affinity antibody producing cells are
preferentially selected to proliferate and in time come to
predominate in the population of cells producing antibody.
Thus, the immune response behaves as a type of microevolu-
tionary system with decreasing antigen concentration acting
as the selective pressure. On the basis of such a
selectional theory for the immune response and the hypothesis
that the mechanism of suppression is the binding of free
antigen by antibody, one can make a number of predictions
which we have tested in our laboratory.

For example, based upon this theoretical framework we
can predict that suppression should be dependent on the
antibody dose. That is, the larger the dose of antibody the
greater the degree of suppression. Similarly one would
predict that the larger the dose of antigen the more antibody would be required to bind it and thus the more passive
antibody would be required for suppression. Furthermore, if
suppression depends upon the binding of antigen then
suppression should be related to the affinity of the passive
antibody. Thus, high affinity passive antibody should be
more effective than low affinity antibody in causing
suppression. Finally, one would predict that as the affinity
of the cell population increases with time after immunization
only higher affinity passive antibody could bring about
suppression. These predictions have all been tested and

found to be true in our laboratory (14,15). The results are
summarized in Tables I-IV and Figure 1. It is of interest to
note in Figure 1 and Table I that a subsuppressive dose of
passive antibody may cause an augmentation of the antibody
response. This is particularly characteristic of high
affinity passive antibody. A similar augmentation of the
antibody response by passive antibody has been observed by
other workers (16,17).

TABLE I

*Effect of Dose of Passive Antibody
on Suppression of the Antibody Response*[*]

Dose Passive Antibody	Antibody Concentration % of Normal	
(mg)	Day 13 (%)	Day 20 (%)
0.6	101	---
2.0	115	145
6.1	44	140
13.5	9	35

[*] *Rabbits received various doses of rabbit
anti-DNP-BGG antibody intravenously one day
before immunizatin with 5 mg DNP-BGG in
complete Freund's adjuvant. Animals were
bled at 13 and 20 days after immunization.
Antibody concentration was determined by
quantitative precipitin reaction using
DNP-bovine fibrinogen as antigen and the
results are presented as percent of antibody
response by animals which received no
passive antibody. Data are adapted from
Walker and Siskind (14) and are averages of
groups of five to 11 rabbits.*

TABLE II

*Effect of Antigen Dose
on Suppression by Passive Antibody**

Antibody Concentration			
0.5 mg DNP-BGG		5.0 mg DNP-BGG	
Normal (mg/ml)	Suppressed (mg/ml)	Normal (mg/ml)	Suppressed (mg/ml)
2.05	0.01	1.78	0.45
3.87	0.03	1.45	1.64
1.99	0.00	0.44	0.10
0.53	0.06	1.62	0.80
0.93	0.00	0.93	0.12
	0.03		0.16
1.87	0.02 Average	1.24	0.55

* *Rabbits received rabbit anti-DNP-BGG antibody
intravenously. They were immunized with the
indicated dose of DNP-BGG in complete Freund's
adjuvant one day later, and were bled three
weeks later. Antibody concentration was
determined by quantitative precipitin reaction
using DNP-bovine fibrinogen as antigen. Data
are from Siskind (15).*

TABLE III

Effect of Antibody Affinity on the Amount
of Passive Antibody Required to
Produce 50% Suppression of Antibody
Synthesis Two Weeks after Immunization[*]

Affinity (K_o) of Passive Antibody (kcal/mole)	Amount of Passive Antibody (mg)
1.9×10^6	49
6.1×10^7	14
1.0×10^{11}	6

[*] *Groups of rabbits received varying doses of*
rabbit anti-DNP-BGG antibody of various
affinities intravneously and were immunized
with 5 mg DNP-BGG in complete Freund's
adjuvant one day later. Animals were bled
two weeks after immunization and the anti-
DNP antibody concentration determined by
quantitative precipitin reaction using
DNP-bovine fibrinogen as antigen. The
amount of passive antibody required for
50% inhibition of antibody synthesis was
calculated and is presented in the table.
The data are derived from Walker and
Siskind (14).

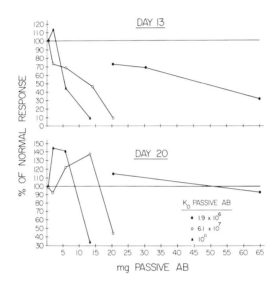

Figure 1. Rabbits received varied doses of anti-
DNP antibody of different affinities. The
animals were immunized one day later with
5 mg DNP-BGG in complete Freund's adjuvant
and were bled 13 and 20 days later. Antibody
concentration was determined by quantitative
precipitin reaction using DNP-bovine fibrinogen
as antigen. The data are expressed as percent
of the response of animals which received no
passive antibody. Each point represents an
average of data obtained on between three and
25 animals (average of nine animals studied
per point). Data are derived from Walker and
Siskind (14).

TABLE IV

*Effect of Antibody Affinity on the Ability of Passive Antibody to Suppress Antibody Synthesis as a Function of Time After Immunization**

| Passive Antibody | | Concentration of Antibody | | | |
| | | Days After Immunization | | | |
Start (day)	Affinity(K_0) (kcal/mole)	15 (mg/ml)	21 (mg/ml)	28 (mg/ml)	35 (mg/ml)
None	----	0.75	1.32	2.47	3.40
1	2×10^6	0.20	----	----	----
8	2×10^6	----	2.14	3.07	----
8	6×10^7	----	0.86	1.53	----
21	6×10^7	----		2.28	2.55
21	1×10^{11}	----		1.67	1.66

* Rabbits were immunized with 0.5 mg DNP-BGG in complete Freund's adjuvant and were injected with 20 mg rabbit anti-DNP-BGG antibody intravenously on the day indicated under "start" and a second injection of 10 mg antibody one week later. The affinity of the passive antibody for DNP-lysine is indicated. The animals were bled on the days indicated and the concentration of antibody determined by quantitative precipitin reaction using DNP-bovine fibrinogen as antigen. Data are extracted from Siskind (15) and represent an average of groups of five to 22 animals.

Carrier specificity is classically associated with T-cell functions such as delayed hypersensitivity. However, it should be recalled that serum antibody also exhibits carrier specificity based upon the fact that the interaction between antigen and antibody involve regions of the antigen molecule in addition to the hapten itself. Thus, we have shown that as much as one-third of the total energy of interaction may be involved in carrier related interactions (18). Based upon these considerations, and the demonstrated affinity dependence of suppression (Table III and Figure 1), I would expect that passive antibody mediated suppression would exhibit significant carrier specificity. As illustrated in Table V, we have found this to be true (19).

As discussed above, the antibody response to the usual haptenic determinants generally consists of a large array of molecules of varying affinity for the hapten. Since available evidence (11,21) suggests that individual B cells produce a homogeneous antibody product this array of anti-body molecules must be reflected in a corresponding array of B lymphocytes. As discussed above, with time after immunization the high affinity components of this array are preferentially selected to proliferate and produce antibody. One can ask what portion of this array would be suppressed preferentially if animals are given passive antibody. Clearly, if passive antibody competes with potential antibody forming cells for available antigen then one would predict that low affinity antibody producing cells would be preferentially suppressed. This would result in an increased affinity of the residual antibody produced. We have found this to be true in several systems (9,22) as illustrated in Table VI and Figure 2. A second effect of suppression on affinity is also illustrated in Figure 2. If the immune response is markedly depressed by any procedure, selection for high affinity antibody synthesis becomes less efficient (24). For efficient selection to occur in any evolving system a marked degree of proliferation is necessary. Thus, with marked suppression one would expect that the selection for high affinity antibody synthesis would be inefficient and the affinity of the residual antibody would be low. This effect of a high dose of passive antibody is illustrated in Figure 2.

TABLE V

Carrier Specificity of Immune Suppression
by Passive Anti-DNP-BGG Antibody*

Anti-DNP-BGG Antibody	Antigen	Direct Anti-DNP PFC		Indirect Anti-DNP PFC	
		PFC/Spleen	Percent Depression (%)	PFC/Spleen	Percent Depression (%)
None	DNP-BGG	6,956	---	46,500	---
+	DNP-BGG	105	98	500	99
None	DNP-RSA	1,500	---	6,940	---
+	DNP-RSA	756	50	8,920	-29

* Groups of mice received normal mouse serum or mouse anti-DNP-BGG anti-serum intravenously one day before immunization with 0.1 mg of either DNP-BGG or DNP-RSA intraperitoneally in complete Freund's adjuvant. The animals were sacrificed one week after immunization and the plaque forming cell response in their spleens assayed against DNP-Ova coated sheep RBC in the Kennedy and Axelrad (20) plaquing system. The data represent geo-metric means of groups of five to seven mice. The data are taken from Birnbaum, Weksler and Siskind (19).

TABLE VI

Effect of Repeated Injections
of Passive Anti-DNP Antibody on the Affinity
of the Anti-DNP Antibody Produced*

Exp.	Passive Antibody	Antibody Concentration (mg/ml)	Antibody Affinity
1	None	1.26 (8)	9.7 (8)
	Anti–DNP	0.39 (6)	10.9 (6)
2	None	0.44 (8)	0.72 (8)
	Anti–BSA	0.03 (8)	0.91 (7)

* *In experiment 1, rabbits received 20 mg*
rabbit anti-DNP-BGG antibody one day before
immunization with 5 mg DNP-BGG in complete
Freund's adjuvant. Repeated injections of
antibody were given at weekly intervals.
Animals were bled 20 days after immunization
and antibody concentration determined by
quantitative precipitin reaction with DNP-
bovine fibrinogen and affinity for DNP-lysine
determined by fluorescence quenching. The
numbers in parentheses indicate the number of
animals studied. Data are from Siskind, Dunn
and Walker (9). In Experiment 2, rabbits were
immunized with 1 mg BSA in complete Freund's
adjuvant one day after they received either
nothing or 20mg rabbit anti-BSA antibody
intravenously. The animals were bled two
weeks after immunization. Antibody concen-
tration was determined by quantitative preci-
pitin reaction with BSA and avidity by the
technique of Celada, Schmidt and Strom (23)
and expressed as the slope of the regression
line. A higher slope indicates greater
avidity. The data are taken from Heller and
Siskind (22).

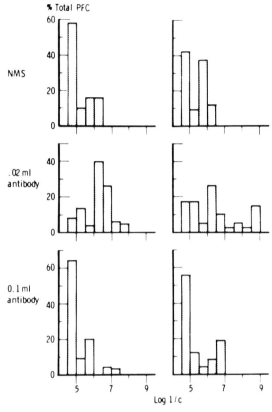

Figure 2. Effect of passive antibody on the distribution of affinity of plaque forming cells. Mice
received either normal mouse serum (NMS), 0.02 ml
or 0.1 ml of mouse anti-DNP-BGG antibody intravenously and were immunized with 0.1 mg DNP-BGG in
complete Freund's adjuvant intraperitoneally one
day later. Animals were sacrificed seven days
after immunization and the distribution of affinities
of the indirect anti-DNP plaque forming cells in
their spleen assayed by inhibition of plaque formation with DNP-EACA in the Kennedy and Axelrad (20)
plaquing system. The percent of total PFC in a given
affinity subpopulation is plotted on the ordinate
against the log of the reciprocal of the hapten
concentration used for inhibition of plaque formation. Affinity increases to the right. Each graph
represents data on an individual mouse. The data
are in part from Birnbaum, Weksler and Siskind (19)
and in part are previously unpublished data of
Birnbaum, Weksler and Siskind.

If, as discussed above, the mechanism of suppression is the binding of the antigenic determinant by antibody thus blocking its interaction with potential antibody-forming cells, then one would expect Fab fragments to be capable of causing suppression. In addition, one would expect suppression to be antigenic determinant specific rather than antigen molecule specific. That is, if one had an antigen with two distinct antigenic determinants (e.g., two haptens coupled to the same carrier molecule) then passive antibody to one determinant would be expected to suppress antibody synthesis to that determinant without depressing the antibody response to the second determinant. In Table VII are presented data indicating that Fab fragments are capable of causing suppression (25). In Table VIII is presented the results of studies on suppression of the antibody response using rabbit gamma globulin substituted with two different, noncross-reactive haptens as antigen (26). It is clear that passive antibody specific for one hapten can suppress the response to that determinant without altering the antibody response to the second hapten. Thus, in this system, suppression is determinant specific as predicted.

An alternative hypothesis for the mechanism of antibody mediated suppression is that antibody molecules specifically inhibit synthesis by those cells making that particular antibody molecule. That is, suppression operates by some type of product mediated feedback inhibition mechanism in which the passive antibody acts directly upon potential antibody forming cells rather than indirectly by interacting with antigen. Most of the data described above is not clearly inconsistent with this hypothesis. Several testable predictions can be derived from the alternative hypothesis. For example, one would expect suppression by high affinity antibody to preferentially inhibit high affinity antibody synthesis and, in contrast, suppression with low affinity antibody would specifically suppress low affinity antibody synthesis. This has been tested and the data obtained are inconsistent with the prediction from this hypothesis (14). A single dose of passive antibody has little or no effect on the affinity of the residual antibody formed. In order to demonstrate the preferential suppression of low affinity antibody as described above, it is generally necessary to have repeated injections of passive antibody so as to obtain a chronically increased selective pressure for selection of high affinity antibody synthesis (Table VI).

TABLE VII

Suppression with Fab   Fragments
of Rabbit Anti-DNP Antibody*

Antibody Concentration	
Normal (mg/ml)	Suppressed (mg/ml)
1.16	0.03
1.18	0.17
1.51	0.00
0.73	
1.15 --Average--	0.07

* *Rabbits were immunized with 5 mg DNP-BGG and*
bled 13 days later. Animals were given
20 mg Fab' antibody fragments intravenously
on the day before immunization and 10 mg daily
for the next nine days. Antibody concentration
was determined by quantitative precipitin
reaction using DNP-bovine fibrinogen as
antigen. The data are from Chang, Schneck,
Brody, Deutsch and Siskind (25).

TABLE VIII

Demonstration of Determinant Specificity of Suppression in Rabbits Immunized with DNP-R-Azo-RGG*

Specificity of Passive Antibody	Day 13		Day 20	
	Anti-DNP (mg/ml)	Anti-R-Azo (mg/ml)	Anti-DNP (mg/ml)	Anti-R-Azo (mg/ml)
None	0.33	0.09	0.47	0.10
Anti-DNP-BGG	0.07	0.12	0.12	0.10
Anti-R-Azo-BGG	0.26	0.05	0.56	0.02

* *Rabbits were given 20 mg of either anti-DNP-BGG or anti-R-Azo-BGG antibody intravenously one day before immunization with 5 mg DNP-R-Azo-BGG in complete Freund's adjuvant. Animals were bled 13 and 20 days later and the concentration of antibody determined by quantitative precipitin reaction using R-Azo-BGG or DNP-bovine fibrinogen as antigen. The data represent averages of groups of 9-15 rabbits. Data are taken from Brody, Walker and Siskind (26).*

A second prediction from this alternative hypothesis of
direct interaction of the circulating antibody with potential
antibody forming cells is that a defined subpopulation of the
antibody molecules (e.g., crossreacting antibody molecules)
should preferentially suppress synthesis of that particular
subpopulation of antibody molecules. We have tested this
prediction in the following system (25). Approximately 30%
of the anti-DNP antibody formed in response to immunization
with DNP-BGG will crossreact with the p-nitro-phenyl hapten
(when assayed by the ability to precipitate p-nitrophenyl-
bovine fibrinogen). Crossreacting antibody was purified and
used to suppress the immune response of rabbits to DNP-BGG.
The percent crossreactive antibody in the suppressed and in
normal animals was determined and found to be identical (25).
The passive crossreactive antibody suppressed the anti-DNP
response without preferentially suppressing the crossreactive
subpopulation of antibody molecules. Thus, the results
(Table IX) are inconsistent with the alternative hypothesis
of a direct effect of antibody on the antibody forming cells.

The data are therefore consistent with the hypothesis
that suppression is the result of antibody binding antigen
and thereby blocking the interaction of the antigenic
determinant with potential antibody forming cells. It should
be noted that there have also been data reported supporting
rapid clearance of opsonized antigen as a second mechanism
of suppression in some cases (27).

The existence of the phenomenon of antibody mediated
suppression raises the question of how one can explain the
possibility of eliciting a secondary response in the presence
of circulating antibody. Furthermore, the progressive
increase in affinity of antibody for several months after
injection of antigen suggests a continued selective effect of
antigen which is exerted even in the presence of significant
amounts of circulating antibody. It should be noted that
while an increase in affinity can be demonstrated when
immunization is accomplished by repeated doses of soluble
antigen (24), the most efficient selection for high affinity
antibody synthesis is seen when Freund's adjuvant is employed
and a depot of antigen is consequently established.

Clearly for selection to proceed, or a secondary
response to be elicited, in the presence of serum antibody

TABLE IX

*Use of Anti-DNP Antibody Eluted
with p-Nitro-Phenyl-ε-Amino-n-Caproic Acid
for Suppression of Anti-DNP Antibody Formed
by Rabbits Immunized with DNP-BGG**

Passive Antibody	Antibody Concentration (mg/ml)	Percent Extracted with p-NP-EACA (percent)
None	1.39 (7)	27 (7)
+	0.35 (6)	30 (6)

*   *Rabbits received nothing or 20 mg of purified
anti-DNP antibody prepared by p-NP-EACA extraction of a specific precipitate of anti-DNP-BGG
antibody with DNP-bovine fibrinogen. Animals
were immunized one day later with 5 mg DNP-BGG
in complete Freund's adjuvant and were bled
two weeks later. The concentration of antibody
was measured by quantitative precipitin
reaction with DNP-bovine fibrinogen. The
percent of the antibody produced which could
be extracted with p-NP-EACA from a specific
precipitate formed at equivalence with DNP-
bovine fibrinogen was determined. The number
of animals studied is indicated in parentheses.
The data are taken from Chang, Schneck, Brody,
Deutsch and Siskind (25).*

requires some explanation. Recent studies (28,29) which we
have carried out in collaboration with Jean-Claude Bystryn
and John Uhr, suggest that with multivalent antigens specific
cells have a significant advantage over serum type antibody
in capturing antigen. The systems studied involve the binding

of monovalent or polyvalent DNP conjugates to MOPC-315 mouse myeloma cells. MOPC-315 is known to secrete an IgA molecule which binds DNP haptens with relatively high affinity. It was shown that a multivalent DNP conjugate binds to cells with an avidity 100 to 300 times greater than that of a univalent conjugate. This increase in affinity can be explained as a consequence of the stabilizing effect of multiple bond formation between the cell associated antibody and antigenic determinants on individual polyvalent antigen molecules. It was further shown that binding of polyvalent antigen to cells could be blocked by anti-DNP antibody. However, anti-DNP antibody was quite inefficient in competing with the highly "polyvalent" cells for the polyvalent DNP conjugate. In effect the anti-DNP antibody appeared to slow the binding of polyvalent antigen to cells but was relatively inefficient in blocking binding of antigen to cells. It can thus be reasonably hypothesized that the formation of multiple bonds between antigen and potential antibody forming cells is responsible for the ability of antigen to stimulate cells even in the presence of signficiant amounts of circulating antibody.

ACKNOWLEDGEMENTS

This work was supported in part by research grants AM-13701 and AI-11694 from the U.S.P.H.S., N.I.H. The author is a Career Scientist of the Health Research Council of the City of New York under Investigatorship I-593.

I would like to thank Miss Antoinette L. Sapienza for secretarial assistance.

REFERENCES

1. Smith, T., J. Exp. Med., *11*: 241, 1909.

2. Uhr, J.W. and Möller, G., Adv. Immunol., *8*: 81, 1968.

3. Graf, M.W. and Uhr, J.W., J. Exp. Med., *130*: 1175, 1969.

4. Bystryn, J.-C., Graf, M.W. and Uhr, J.W., J. Exp. Med., *132*: 1279, 1970.

5. Pollack, W., Gorman, J.G., Freda, V.J., Ascari, W.Q., Allen, A.E. and Baker, W.J., Transfusion, *8*: 151, 1968.

6. Ascari, W.Q. and Pollack, W., In this symposium, 1975.

7. Karush, F., Adv. Immunol., *2*: 1, 1962.

8. Eisen, H.N. and Siskind, G.W., Biochemistry, *3*: 996, 1964.

9. Siskind, G.W., Dunn, P. and Walker, J.G., J. Exp. Med., *127*: 55, 1968.

10. Goidl, E.A., Paul, W.E., Siskind, G.W. and Benacerraf, B., J. Immunol., *100*: 371, 1968.

11. Siskind, G.W. and Benacerraf, B., Adv. Immunol., *10*: 1, 1969.

12. Werblin, T.P. and Siskind, G.W., Transplant. Rev., *8*: 104 1972.

13. Burnet, F.M., *The Clonal Selection Theory of Immunity*, Vanderbilt and Cambridge University Presses, London and New York, 1959.

14. Walker, J.G. and Siskind, G.W., Immunology, *14*: 21, 1968.

15. Siskind, G.W., in *Developmental Aspects of Antibody Formation and Structure*, Edited by Sterzl, J. and Riha, I., Vol. II, p. 837, Academic Press, New York, 1969.

16. Morrison, S.L. and Terres, G., J. Immunol., *96*: 901, 1966.

16a. Pincus, C.S., Lamm, M.E. and Nussenzweig, V., J. Exp.
      Med., *133*: 987, 1971.

17.   Pollack, W., Gorman, J.G., Hager, H.J., Freda, V.J. and
      Tripodi, D., Transfusion, *8*: 134, 1968.

18.   Paul, W.E., Siskind, G.W. and Benacerraf, B., J. Exp.
      Med., *123*: 689, 1966.

19.   Birnbaum, G., Weksler, M.E. and Siskind, G.W., J. Exp.
      Med., *141*: 411, 1975.

20.   Kennedy, J.C. and Axelrad, M.A., Immunology, *20*: 252,
      1971.

21.   Klinman, N.R., Immunochemistry, *6*: 757, 1969.

22.   Heller, K.S. and Siskind, G.W., Cell. Immunol., *6*: 59,
      1973.

23.   Celada, F., Schmidt, D. and Strom, R., Immunology,
      17: 189, 1969.

24.   Mond, J., Kim, Y.T. and Siskind, G.W., J. Immunol.,
      112: 1255, 1974.

25.   Chang, H., Schneck, S., Brody, N.I., Deutsch, A. and
      Siskind, G.W., J. Immunol., *102*: 37, 1969.

26.   Brody, N.I., Walker, J.G. and Siskind, G.W., J. Exp.
      Med., *126*: 81, 1967.

27.   Klapper, J.W., van der Hoven, A., Dharmarojan, U. and
      Hoffman, M., J. Immunol., *111*: 1228, 1973.

28.   Bystryn, J.-C., Siskind, G.W. and Uhr, J.W., J. Exp.
      Med., *137*: 301, 1973.

29.   Bystryn, J.-C., Siskind, G.W. and Uhr, J.W., J. Exp.
      Med., In press.

DISCUSSION FOLLOWING PRESENTATION

by DR. GREGORY W. SISKIND

R. SHANDAR: Is antibody mediated suppression involved in the immune response to leukemia associated antigens?

G. SISKIND: Perhaps Dr. Good would like to comment in response to that question?

R. GOOD: I don't feel that there is sufficient data available to answer that question adequately.

Z. OVARY: You described mainly effects on the IgG antibody response. Is it also possible to suppress IgM synthesis?

G. SISKIND: I haven't specifically studied IgM responses. However, studies by other laboratories would indicate that it is also possible to suppress IgM antibody synthesis. As I recall the data, there are some systems where one can elicit an IgM response with lower doses of antigen than are required to elicit IgG antibody synthesis. Under such circumstances, it seems to require more passive antibody to suppress IgM synthesis than IgG synthesis.

It might also be noted that IgM antibody can be employed to cause suppression. However, it appears as if, in low doses, IgM antibodies have a distinct tendency to cause an augmentation of the immune response. This is also true for IgG antibody. As I showed earlier, passive IgG antibodies, especially of high affinity, when given in subsuppressive doses can cause a significant augmentation of the immune response. As shown by work of Nussenzweig and of Pollack, this augmentation is not determinant specific, but effects other antigenic determinants on the same molecule.

Some work has suggested that IgM antibodies have a
greater tendency to cause such augmentation than do
IgG antibodies. The mechanism of augmentation is not
understood. Perhaps it involves aggregation of the
antigen to facilitate its favorable localization.

L. WASHINGTON: Is antibody mediated suppression reversible?
    Do repeated doses of passive antibody and antigen lead
    to tolerance induction?

G. SISKIND: Antibody mediated suppression is totally
    reversible. When the passive antibody disappears as a
    result of normal metabolic processes the suppressive
    effect vanishes. Tolerance has never been reported as
    a consequence of antibody mediated suppression.
    However, the observations of Feldmann that antigen-
    antibody complexes, in appropriate ratios, can induce
    tolerance *in vitro* does raise the possibility that such
    an effect might occur *in vivo*. However, the relatively
    narrow ratio of antigen to antibody over which
    tolerance is induced *in vitro* suggests that tolerance
    induction by such a mechanism *in vivo* would be highly
    unlikely. How do you feel about this Dr. Katz?

D. KATZ: I would agree with your answer.

I. SIEGEL: Why do cells bind antigen more effectively than
    does serum antibody? Is there a heterogeneity of
    binding properties among the T-cell population
    comparable to that present in the B-cell population.

G. SISKIND: The formation of multiple bonds between an
    individual multivalent antigen molecule and the cell
    surface leads to a marked augmentation of the energy of
    of interaction. Essentially if two independent bonds
    are formed between the antigen molecule and the cell
    surface, then for the complex to dissociate both bonds
    must dissociate simultaneously. Under such conditions
    the probability of dissociation of the complex becomes
    the product of the probabilities of the dissociation
    of the individual bonds. That is, for both bonds to
    dissociate simultaneously is a very improbable event.

Thus, formation of multiple bonds between an individual, multivalent, antigen molecule and the cell surface would tend to stabilize the complex and make dissociation of the antigen molecule extremely unlikely. The stabilizing effect of multiple bond formation is the essential reason why binding of antigen to the cell surface is favored over binding to serum antibody.

In regard to your second question, very little is known about the binding properties of T lymphocytes for antigen. Thus, it is not possible to say if there is an array of T cells comparable to the array of B cells with respect to affinity for the antigenic determinant.

E. JOHNSON: Can passive antibody turn off antibody synthesis by a cell which is already synthesizing antibody?

G. SISKIND: I do not really know the answer to that question. Perhaps Dr. Wigzell has some information?

H. WIGZELL: I have shown that passive antibody can turn off an ongoing immune response. It takes about 40 hours after administration of the passive antibody to turn off active antibody producing cells.

R. GERHSON: Why do you think it is harder to suppress primed as compared with naive T cells as I discussed earlier today?

G. SISKIND: I really do not know how to answer that question. The number and affinity of antigen binding sites on the population of primed as compared with naive T cells is not known. Thus, it is really impossible to logically arrive at any conclusions. One might mention that it appears to require less antigen to trigger a secondary response as compared with a primary response. This of course is consistent with the greater difficulty of suppressing a secondary response, but does not explain the mechanisms involved.

Rh IMMUNE SUPPRESSION: RE-EXAMINED

William Q. Ascari and William Pollack

Somerset Hospital, Somerville, New Jersey
and
Ortho Diagnostic Research Foundation, Raritan, New Jersey

INTRODUCTION

Almost 15 years have passed since the first human volunteer studies on Rh immune suppression were conceived and implemented. In that interval, literally thousands of volunteers have been studied prospectively in carefully controlled studies. The safety, specificity and efficacy of Rh immune suppression in the prevention of maternal Rh_o (D) isoimmunization by pregnancy has been established beyond doubt. Fortunately, the successful application of this type of immune suppression is undiminished by our as yet incomplete understanding of its mechanism. We maintain an ongoing academic interest in this immunologic model not only for its practical application but for the insight it provides into the mechanism of immune induction in the hope of gleaning still more clues to that central mystery. To that end, we have re-examined the results of several of our previous studies.

RESULTS AND DISCUSSION

The first Rh immune suppression studies in this country which were performed on Rh_o (D) negative inmate volunteers. It demonstrated that Rh_o (D) isoimmunization could be prevented by an "excess of anti-Rh_o (D)". In those studies

115

(1), the "antibody excess" was 4,000-6,000 µg anti-Rh$_O$ (D) administered within 72 hours after 2 ml of Rh$_O$ (D) positive cells. Even before the first studies were completed, it was obvious that the amount of antibody employed was far in excess of that which was actually required. For example, treated volunteers often demonstrated passive Rh$_O$ (D) immunization nine to 12 months following their last injections of immune globulin.

Further testing in Rh$_O$ (D) negative male volunteers revealed that the dose of antibody could be reduced to approximately 5% of the original amount while still obtaining complete Rh$_O$ (D) immune suppression (2). It was shown that 300 µg of anti-Rh$_O$ (D) was "sufficient excess" to prevent immunization of Rh negative volunteers given 10 ml of Rh positive blood. At these levels of antibody and antigen, circulating passive antibody could be demonstrated rarely and then only for short periods after injection.

"Antibody excess" is a relative term - that is, relative to the immunogenicity of its corresponding antigen. The Rh$_O$ (D) antigen is several orders of magnitude less immunogenic than the heterologous antigens commonly employed in immunologic studies in lower animals. It would seem, therefore, that immune suppression to the Rh antigen should be correspondingly easier to achieve (3). While the 300 µg dose appeared to be 100% effective for volumes of Rh positive blood up to 10 ml and was the dosage ultimately selected for prevention of maternal isoimmunization by pregnancy, an additional study was planned using much lower doses of antibody. In this study (4), previously unimmunized Rh$_O$ (D) negative male volunteers were given injections of 5 ml of Rh$_O$ (D) positive blood. They were then given intramuscular injections from coded vials containing 0, 1 µg, 10 µg, 20 µg, and 40 µg of anti-Rh$_O$ (D). The volunteers were tested at monthly intervals for six months when they were given a 0.2 ml injection of Rh$_O$ (D) positive cells as a booster. Final testing was performed two weeks later. The results are shown in Table I.

Forty-nine volunteers were available at the completion of the study. In none of the five groups was there evidence of immune suppression to Rh obtained. At least one group (10 µg) showed evidence of possible augmentation - that is,

TABLE I

The Effect of Low Doses of IgG Anti-Rh (D)-Containing Human Immune Globulin on the Immune Response to 5 ml of Rh Positive Blood

		Dose of Rh Immune Globulin			
	0*	1 μg	10 μg	20 μg	40 μg
Number immunized to Rh / Number studied	1/6	4/13	8/11	3/12	2/10
Percent responding	16.7	30.8	72.7	25	20

* *Control group given immune globulin free of Rh antibodies. The values for responses in each group do not differ significantly from one to the other (0.1 < P < 0.25).*

the percentage of immunized subjects was higher than that observed in the control group. This impression, although not statistically confirmed due to the small number of subjects tested, is strengthened by the finding of multiple blood group antibodies in addition to anti-D in the sera of four of the eight volunteers immunized.

Although the phenomena of immune augmentation might have been anticipated from previous work (5), it confirmed our greatest fears. Finn *et al.* had reported (6) a similar paradoxical response in their experimental Rh immune suppression. They employed whole human serum having a high titer of anti-D. These authors recognized the phenomenon of immune augmentation only in retrospect and then attributed it to the IgM anti-D known to be present in the hyperimmune serum. Immune augmentation was considered to be a particular danger at that time since: (a) Quantitation of the D antigenic stimulus was not routinely performed. A fixed dose of anti-D might prove the augmentation favoring ratio for an unanticipated large feto-maternal hemorrhage. (b) The red cell has more than 100 recognized antigens, most of which are extremely poor immunogens. If production of multiple blood group antibodies did occur as a result of the immune augmentation, it might preclude the possibility of future homologous blood transfusion.

In our study, the volunteers suspected of showing an augmented immune response were carefully studied serologically as shown in Table II. In addition to the multiplicity of blood group antibodies found in some cases, two other peculiarities are to be noted: (a) In no case did multiple blood group antibodies occur in which anti-D did not also appear. (b) IgM anti-D antibodies persisted for a much longer duration than is normally observed with Rh immune induction. This may reflect a delay in the production of IgG anti-Rh$_o$ (D).

Serologically, evidence of Rh immune augmentation is present in all of the eight immunized volunteers in the 10 µg group and two of the three immunized volunteers in the 1 µg and 40 µg groups showed these serologic properties. This is a remarkable narrow range of antibody-antigen ratio for immune augmentation if indeed the phenomena of augmentation represents the adjuvant properties of blood group

antibodies in concentrations that are too low to achieve
suppression.

Since the very low dose study had failed to demonstrate
the minimal antibody-antigen ratio required for Rh immune
suppression, we embarked upon still another study in which
the variable was the amount of the D antigen administered
(7). Two hundred two Rh_O (D) negative volunteers with no
history of exposure to or serologic evidence of immunization
by the Rh_O (D) antigen were given intravenous injections of
Rh_O (D) positive blood varying from 25-100 ml. One-half of
the volunteers served as controls and subsequently received
an intramuscular injection of immune globulin containing no
anti-Rh. The other half of the volunteers were treated with
intramuscular injections of immune globulin containing
267 μg anti-Rh_O (D) positive blood. Final serologic testing
was performed two weeks later. The results are shown on
Table III.

In assembling this data, it was apparent that the
volume of Rh_O (D) positive blood injected should be expressed
as ml of packed cells to correct for the differences in the
hematocrit of the donor blood. Accordingly, six groups were
formed each with its treated and control subjects from the
178 volunteers who completed the study. Rh_O (D) immune suppression was completely successfully in the first two groups
(i.e. those receiving an average of 11.6 ml and 13.4 ml of
Rh_O positive blood as packed cells). A progressive "escape"
from complete suppression was noted in the remaining four
"treated" groups who presumably received an inadequate amount
of anti-D relative to the dose of D antigen injected.
Despite the inadequate dosage of specific antibody, no immune
augmentation was observed.

The data from Table III have been illustrated graphically in Figure 1 to show the relationship between the treated
and the control groups. As the volume of Rh_O (D) positive
cells injected increases the probability of immunization
rises. The ordinate value to be expected from an infinitely
large volume of blood was found to be 36% for the treated
group and 68% for the control group. The extrapolated value
for the control group appears to be valid since not all
individuals appear to have the same susceptibility to Rh_O (D)
isoimmunization. By contrast, the extrapolation for the

TABLE II

Class and Specificity of the Antibody Response in Male Volunteers given Low Doses of Anti-Rh$_o$ (D) Containing Immune Globulin

Group	No. Immunized to Rh Number studied	Volunteer	Type of Anti-Rh$_o$ (D) Response	Other Red Cell Antibodies
Control	1/6	H.S.	IgG only	None
1 μg	4/13	M.K.	IgG only	None
		R.R.	IgG only	None
		G.S.	IgG only	None
		J.M.	IgG only	None
10 μg	8/11	R.Br.	IgM* later IgG	None
		R.R.	IgM later IgG	None
		E.DeR.	IgM later IgG	None
		R.N.	IgM later IgG	Anti-E, anti-S
		R.Bn.	IgG only	Anti-E
		M.S.	IgM later IgG	None
		R.M.	IgM later IgG	Anti-E, anti-JK[a]
		G.S.	IgM later IgG	Unidentified antibodies

120

20 µg	3/12	P.M.	IgM later IgG	Anti-E, anti-JK[a]
		J.S.	IgM later IgG	None
		D.G.	IgG only	None
40 µg	2/10	F.H.	IgG only	None
		J.Sp.	IgG only	None

* *IgM antibody response was judged by agglutination of saline suspended cells and sensitivity to 0.1 M 2-mercaptoethanol.*

TABLE III

Incidence of Rh Immunization in Rh Negative Volunteers
Receiving Different Quantities of Rh Positive Blood*

Group:	A	B	C	D	E	F
Cell Volume[+]:	11.6	13.4	18.1	21.2	30.1	37.5
(Range)	(10.9-12.4)	(12.6-14.6)	(16.6-19.6)	(20.8-21.3)	(28.4-32.3)	(35.9-41.7)
Treated[§]:	0/19 (0%)	0/18 (0%)	3/18 (16.7%)	2/8 (25%)	4/12 (33.3%)	6/17 (35.3%)
Control[Ψ]:	7/16 (43.8%)	6/12 (50%)	11/19 (57.9%)	5/8 (62.5%)	7/11 (63.6%)	13/20 (65%)

* Results are given as the number of subjects who were successfully Rh immunized divided by the number of subjects in the group. The percent responding to the Rh antigen is given in parentheses.

+ Average packed cell volume (in milliliters) of Rh positive cells injected. The range of doses given to each group is given in parentheses.

§ Each treated volunteer received one vial of Rh immune globulin (ORF Lot CH 862) containing 267 µg anti-Rh_O (D).

Ψ Each control volunteer received one vial of immune globulin (ORF Lot 03) devoid of anti-Rh_O (D).

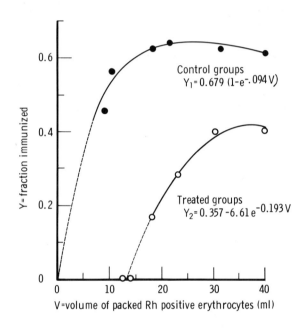

Figure 1. Fraction of male volunteers immunized (Y) for various doses of packed Rh positive red cells (V). Control groups received globulin devoid of anti-Rh$_O$ (D). Treated groups received one vial of immune globulin containing 267 µg anti-Rh$_O$ (D).

treated group can be argued to be invalid for two reasons:
(a) it does not accommodate the phenomenon of augmentation
and (b) it states that even an inadequate dose of anti-Rh
will decrease the probability of isoimmunization irrespective
of the volume of blood injected. If the extrapolation for
the experimental groups were shown to be correct, it would
represent a powerful argument for passively administered
antibody acting on a central processing mechanism rather
than on the immunogen itself. The critical experiment to
establish or refute this point is currently being performed.

The data from the male volunteer study can be linearized
by logarithmic transformation. The regression equation
which satisfactorily describes the data is:

$$y = A - Be^{-cv}$$

where A is the asymptotic value and B and C are constants.
For the Y1 (control) series, B = A since the regression
line must pass through the origin. Logarithmic transformation of the data are shown in Figure 2. As expected,
extrapolation of the data passes through the origin and the
points fall nicely along the linear regression line.

Logarithmic transformation of the data from the Y2
(treated) series is shown in Figure 3. The linear
regression line intercepts the abscissa at a value of
15.1 ml. This represents the maximum volume of Rh positive
red cells which can be neutralized by the 267 µg of anti-Rh$_o$
(D).

We had the opportunity of confirming this hypothesis
in the course of stability studies in which three different
lots of Rh$_o$ (D) immune globulin, each containing
approximately 300 µg anti-Rh$_o$ (D) per dose, were given to Rh
negative males who had previously received intravenous
injections of 15 ml of Rh positive red cells. None of the
52 volunteers became immunized as determined by booster
stimulation six months later (8).

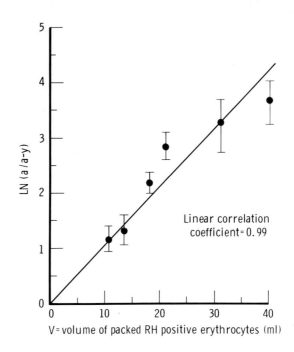

Figure 2. Control series. Linear transformation of Y_1 (control groups) in which

$$Ln \left(\frac{a}{a-y}\right) = cv: \quad a = 0.679 \text{ and } C = 0.094.$$

The 95% confidence limits are indicated in the graph.

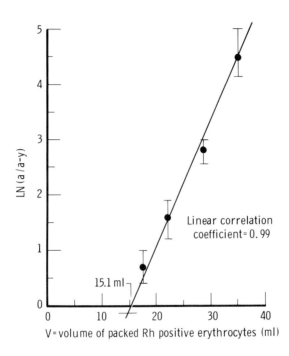

Figure 3. Treated series. Linear transformation of Y_2 (groups treated with anti-Rh_o (D)) in which

$$\text{Ln} \left(\frac{a}{a-y}\right) = \ln \left(\frac{a}{b}\right) + cv:$$

a = 0.357, b = 6.610 and c = 0.193.

The 95% confidence intervals are indicated in the graph.

Turning now to a consideration of molecular events which occur in the Rh negative volunteer being suppressed or augmented by passive immunization. Under *in vitro* conditions, IgG anti-Rh_O (D) antibodies do not agglutinate Rh_O (D) positive erythrocytes and thus behave as if they are serologically monovalent with respect to binding.

The following is the Mass-Law equation that satisfied the binding of anti-Rh positive erythrocytes (Sips absorption isotherm)

$$K_O^\alpha = \frac{\{Ag\ Ab\}}{\{Ag\}^\alpha \{Ab\}}$$

$\{AgAb\}$ = equilibrium concentration of bound antibody (or antigen).

$\{Ag\}$ = equilibrium free antigen concentration = $(T - \{AgAb\})$.

$\{Ab\}$ = equilibrium free antibody concentration = $(N - \{AgAb\})$.

α = index of heterogeneity (α = >0<1).

K_O = average intrinsic binding constant.

N = starting antibody concentration.

T = starting antigen concentration.

At equilibrium, the amount of antibody bound to red cells is determined by five independent variables. These are:

1. The average binding affinity of the antibodies.

2. The number of antibody molecules capable of binding antigen.

3. The number of antigen molecules capable of being bound.

4. The volume in which the antibody is distributed.

5. The volume in which the antigen is distributed.

We will discuss each of these briefly:

The average binding affinity is a numerical expression for the strength of the noncovalent bonding between antibody and antigen. It is the ratio of bound to unbound antibody at equilibrium for any concentration of antigen. Most lots of Rh_o (D) immune globulin prepared from plasma of hyper-immunized donors have an average binding affinity of $1-2 \times 10^8$ liters/mole.

When we speak of the number of antibody molecules capable of binding antigen, we are essentially referring to the total amount of antibody injected since there is no evidence for significant biological attrition in the time frame we are considering. The amount of antibody is quantitated by radioimmunoassay as described previously (9).

Quantitation of the D antigen sites on Rh positive red cells is also performed by radioimmunoassay. We have performed numerous assays on red cells of varying Rh pheno-types and find that 300 picomoles/ml of red cells is a satisfactory average.

We initially considered the volume elements for the red cells and antibodies to the three liters and six liters respectively. The red cells would be confined to the intra-vascular space whereas the antibodies would be equally distributed between the intravascular and extracellular fluid compartments. While this calculation may represent the volume element shortly after the time of injection, it bears no resemblance to the conditions at the time of equilibrium.

As the Rh positive cells circulate in a subject who has anti-D activity, antibody will be bound to no more than 1-2% of the available antigen sites. Since Rh antibodies are uniformly non-complement fixing, lysis does not occur. Instead, red cells lightly coated by antibody are captured by the sieving action of the spleen and thus progressively concentrate within a volume approximating the volume of the white pulp of the spleen. This mass of immobilized red cells is continuously bathed in plasma containing unbound antibody. The Rh_o (D) positive cells will act as an immune absorbant until the volume element for the antibody approaches that of the red cells.

We have utilized these variables in the Mass Law equation to determine the percentage of available antigen which is bound by antibody for each group of male volunteers in two of the studies discussed earlier. The results of our calculations are shown on Table IV. As was noted above, complete immune suppression was achieved by 267 µg anti-Rh_o (D) in treated volunteers who received 11.6 and 13.4 ml of Rh_o (D) positive cells. At a molecular level, we calculate this to represent binding of 30% or more of the available D antigen. According to the calculations, binding to between 13 and 24% of the antigen is sufficient only to reduce the probability of immune induction but not to abolish it in all individuals.

By contrast, our calculations in the case of Rh_o (D) negative volunteers who received 10 or 20 µg anti-D after 5 ml of Rh_o (D) positive cells indicate that the percentage of antigen binding was only 2-3%. This amount of surface antibody might augment the immune response by serving to efficiently concentrate the antigen within the spleen but represents too sparce a density to retard or prevent recognition.

Our calculation that immune suppression occurs when 30% or more of the available antigen is bound very closely approximates the immune suppression results of Uhr and Bauman (3). They observed complete immune suppression when 25-50% of the antigen was bound in diphtheria toxin-rabbit antitoxin studies. We can only conclude that perhaps the difference in immunogenicity between the two antigens is less than anticipated.

TABLE IV

Calculation of Percent of Bound Antigen at Equilibrium

Vol. Packed Rh$_0$ (D) Red Cells Injected (ml)	Final Rh$_0$ (D) Antigen Concentration (M/L)	Final Anti-Rh$_0$ Concentration (M/L)	% of Total Antigen Bound
11.6	3.48×10^{-8}	1.66×10^{-8}	33.5%
13.4	4.02×10^{-8}	1.66×10^{-8}	30.6%
18.1	5.43×10^{-8}	1.66×10^{-8}	24.7%
21.2	6.36×10^{-8}	1.66×10^{-8}	21.9%
30.1	9.03×10^{-8}	1.66×10^{-8}	16.3%
37.5	11.25×10^{-8}	1.66×10^{-8}	13.4%
5.0	2.0×10^{-8}	6.6×10^{-10}	2.2%
5.0	2.0×10^{-8}	13.2×10^{-10}	3.0%

M/L = moles/liter

REFERENCES

1. Freda, V.J., Gorman, J.G. and Pollack, W., Transfusion, *4*: 26, 1964.

2. Pollack, W., Singher, H.O., Gorman, J.G. and Freda, V.J., Hematologia, *2*: 1, 1968.

3. Uhr, J.W. and Bauman, J.B., J. Exp. Med., *113*: 1935, 1901.

4. Pollack, W., Gorman, J.G., Hager, H.J., Freda, V.J. and Tripodi, D., Transfusion, *8*: 134, 1968.

5. Adler, F.L., J. Immunol., *76*: 217, 1956.

6. Finn, R., Clarke, C.A., Donohoe, W.T.A., McConnell, R.B., Sheppard, P.M., Lehane, D. and Kulke, W., Brit. Med. J., *1*: 1486, 1961.

7. Pollack, W., Ascari, W.Q., Kochesky, R.J., O'Connor, R.R., Ho, T.Y. and Tripodi, D., Transfusion, *11*: 333, 1971.

8. Pollack, W. and Ascari, W.Q., Unpublished observations.

9. Pollack, W. and Kochesky, R.J., Int. Arch. Allergy, *38*: 320, 1970.

DISCUSSION FOLLOWING PRESENTATION

by DR. WILLIAM Q. ASCARI

R. GOOD: What is the effect of splenectomy on suppression?
Would you predict from your work that the spleen is
essential for immune suppression?

W. ASCARI: We have not studied any splenectomized subjects.
One problem is we are dealing with an antigen of intermediate immunogenicity.   Even if we administer as much
as 100 ml of red cells, only 60 or 70% of the subjects
are immunized.   Thus, it is necessary to study a large
number of male subjects to arrive at any conclusions.

There is relatively little antigen localized in liver
in patients who are effectively immune suppressed.

I would like to digress a moment if I may. The question
has come up as to the effectiveness of IgM antibodies as
compared with IgG in suppression. On a molecule for
molecule basis I think that they are equally effective,
if one considers equal affinity of binding. I do not
think that IgM predisposes to immune augmentation except
on that basis. I think it tends to give you lower
binding rather than to form precipitates which are
intrinsically more immunogenic. At least, in the studies
of Kim immune augmentation was in the critical range of
2 to 3% rather than up around 30%.

R. GOOD: Have experiments been done to determine if the
spleen has a critical role in the immunosuppressive
effects of antibody?

G. SISKIND: I do not know of any such studies. Dr. Wigzell,
do you know of any studies bearing on this issue?

H. WIGZELL: No, I do not.

O'REILLY: Is there a difference between mixing the antibody
    and antigen prior to injection as compared to giving the
    antigen and antibody separately and allowing them to
    react *in vivo?*

W. ASCARI: We have not tried that experiment.   I presume
    that the antigen-antibody complex will dissociate and
    form a new equilibrium if the dose is inadequate to give
    us an ultimate 30%.

O'REILLY: The real question is whether the interaction of
    the antibody is only with the antigen.   There are also
    possible tissue receptors for antibody and for antigen-
    antibody aggregates.

W. ASCARI: A third of the injected antibody is not bound to
    injected antigen even at equilibrium so it will certainly
    compete for antigen and with antigen for other binding
    sites.

NATURAL IMMUNOSUPPRESSIVE FACTORS

Sidney R. Cooperband, A.H. Glasgow and J.A. Mannick

Departments of Medicine, Microbiology and Surgery,
Cancer Research Center, Boston University School of Medicine
Boston, Massachusetts 02118

INTRODUCTION

The observation that extracts of tissues and fluids of natural origin contain pharmacologically active substances has, historically, been a frequent starting place for the discovery of new biological and physiological processes. Although the concept of suppressor activities in immune reactions did not develop directly in this sequence, it is true that the demonstration of suppressive factors in the serum and lymphoid tissues preceded the current interest in the cellular aspects of immunosuppression by many years. We would like to review the current state of knowledge about these natural humoral immunosuppressive substances, and discuss in more detail the serum immunosuppressive material studied in our laboratories for the past seven to eight years. Collectively, the many publications relating to natural immunosuppressive factors support the idea that there exists within the body, a number of humoral immuno-inhibitory substances which may act non-specifically to antagonize one or another part of the immune response without regard to antigen. Some of these factors act selectively on T cells, some on B cells, and some on macrophages. Most factors are extracted from or produced by lymphoid tissues, but some are found in serum, placenta or amniotic fluid. Many appear to be produced as part of the host normal immune response.

Negative effects by any pharmacologic substance are always subject to some suspicion. It is therefore essential to demonstrate that any immunosuppressive phenomenon produced by natural substances is related only to immunity, and not related to non-specific toxicity, proteolysis or other enzymatic degradation, or to metabolic antagonism. For the most part, the factors to be discussed in this manuscript meet the criteria of being non-specifically immunosuppressive yet without appreciable inhibitory or toxic effects on non-lymphoid cells and tissues. They appear to have selective negative effects upon immune reactivity. The inhibitory effects of these substances are not induced to any specific antigen, nor are they antigen specific in their activity. We will not review the growing list of pharmaceutical agents and exogenous viral products which have suppressive activity, or the many reports which have demonstrated that unfractionated plasma/serum from a variety of clinical disorders may suppress one or another *in vitro* assay of lymphocyte function.

Kamrin, in 1958 (1), was the first to observe that a substance in the serum could inhibit immunity; he found that rat plasma proteins, Cohn Fraction IV, were capable of preserving the parabiotic union of random bred rats. In 1963 Mowbray (2) confirmed these experiments and extended them by fractionating bovine α-globulin fractions on anion-exchange chromatography columns and separating a fraction which could prolong skin allografts. He then demonstrated that this fraction of α-globulin was also immunosuppressive in mice, as measured by an inhibition of antibody production against sheep erythrocytes (3). Neither investigator found any evidence of cytotoxicity in animals receiving these plasma fractions, and both found the suppression was most easily effected when the factor was administered prior to, or simultaneously with antigen.

Our group at Boston University first because involved in this problem in 1967 (4), at which time we successfully repeated Mowbray's work using human plasma as a source of the suppressor factor. We were able to isolate a fraction by DEAE column chromatography of whole fresh human plasma, and demonstrated that this fraction was able to cause significant prolongation of skin allografts in mice across a strong H2 barrier when administered 24-48 hours prior to grafting. This immunosuppression occurred without any evidence of cyto-toxicity in the recipient mice.

Since that time, a number of laboratories around the
world have demonstrated immunosuppressive activity in various
fractions of the serum proteins. Table II presents a brief
summary of those publications that utilized immunosuppressive
fractions from the serum or plasma.

In most cases, the active fractions were those which
contained predominantly α-globulins. Active fractions have
been obtained from the plasmas of rat, cow, guinea pig,
rabbit, mouse and human. For the most part, they have been
suppressive in both the species of origin, and across species
lines. These fractions have been assayed with a variety of
methods, ranging from prolongation of skin allografts to
inhibition of antibody formation; in general, all assays have
required participation of T lymphocytes. The various
fractions have been active at a number of doses, but
generally within the dose range of 0.5-10 mg/ml of extracellular fluid.

IN VITRO STUDIES ON SERUM SUPPRESSORS

In 1968 (5), we discovered that our α-globulin fractions
could prevent the activation of blood lymphocytes induced by
phytohemagglutinin and other mitogens in cell culture. We
found that the human α-globulin could also antagonize the
"blast" transformation (and its attendant increase in protein
and DNA synthesis) of human blood lymphocytes induced by a
variety of antigens to which the donor was sensitive: these
included diphtheria toxoid, tetanus toxoid, tuberculin,
keyhole limpet hemocyaninin, and mixed lymphocyte reactions.
The dose-response curves of suppression with the α-globulin
preparations were unusual. The inhibition of cell activation
occurred over a very narrow dose range (1-2 mg/ml of extracellular fluid), so that the phenomenon is essentially an all
or none type of response. Also, we found that the dose
necessary to inhibit activation varied with the intensity of
the stimulus, i.e., we needed a four-fold higher concentration of α-globulin to antagonize the intense stimulation of
lymphocytes that occurs with PHA than was needed to produce
a similar antagonism of proliferation induced by a mixed
leukocyte culture. Figure 1 demonstrates these effects.

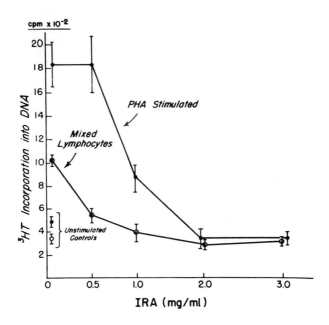

Figure 1. Dose dependent suppression by serum
α-globulin suppressor (IRA) of human blood
lymphocyte stimulation induced by phytohemagglutinin (PHA) and allogeneic cells *in vitro*.
Stimulation of cells estimated by determining
the rate of ³H-thymidine (³HT) incorporation
into acid insoluble DNA during the last 24
hours or a six day culture for PHA stimulated
cells, and a three day culture for the mixed
leukocytes.

    During this time we carried out a large number of
control experiments to demonstrate that this inhibitor of
cell proliferation was specific to lymphocytes, rather than
a general or artifactual antagonist of any cell proliferation.
We demonstrated that the α-globulins did not destroy
essential metabolites, nor did they contrain amino acid (or
other) hydrolases. Examination with trypan-blue indicated
that neither lymphocytes nor a variety or other cells in

tissue culture were damaged by exposure to the α-globulin. The α-globulins did not bind the mitogens or antigens. Studies of the effect of the α-globulin fractions on plating efficiency and growth rate of non-lymphoid cells demonstrated either no effect, or enhanced growth rate and plating efficiency (5).

STUDIES ON THE MECHANISM OF ACTION OF THE SERUM SUPPRESSORS

Using *in vitro* assay systems, we also began to determine how the α-globulin fractions affected the immune response. Experimental results indicated that inhibition of lymphocyte proliferation could occur only when immunocytes were exposed to the α-globulin early in the sequence of the metabolic events leading to lymphocyte activation. Figure 2 illustrates the results of an experiment in which PHA was used to stimulate blood lymphocytes and the time sequence of protein synthesis determined subsequent to PHA activation. The α-globulin fraction was added to one set of cultures at the initiation of the experiment, and to another set   48 hours after the initiation of the experiment. The lymphocytes exposed to the α-globulin from the onset of stimulation were not activated; the lymphocytes exposed to α-globulin after activation of the cells were not inhibited. The latter cultures, moreover, acted as if the mitogen had been removed from the culture, and on the next cell cycle their rate of protein synthesis dropped to that of the unstimulated control. Thus, the α-globulin could antagonize lymphocytes early in the activation of the cell cycle, but had no effect upon metabolic events once the initial activation had occurred (6,7).

In vivo experimentation using sheep erythrocytes (SRBC) in mice later confirmed this conclusion (35). It was observed that administration of the α-globulin at any time (greater than one hour) following antigen failed to prevent a normal primary antibody plaque forming cell response. This serum factor appeared to antagonize some early metabolic event in lymphocyte activation both *in vitro* and *in vivo*; its failure to act later is further proof of the absence of non-specific cytotoxicity or general cytostasis.

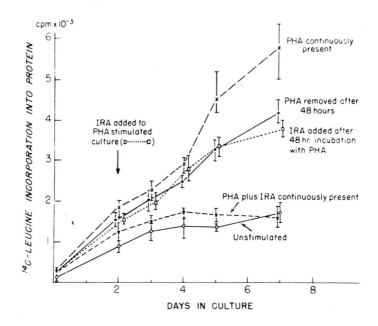

Figure 2. Addition of suppressor α-globulin (IRA)
to human blood lymphocyte cultures after
activation by PHA. "Activation" estimated by
the rate of ^{14}C-leucine incorporation into
protein determined serially for seven days.

Using washed blood lymphocytes we were able to absorb
small quantities of α-globulin suppressor activity from
standardized solutions (7). The suppressive effect of the
α-globulin appeared to be easily removed, however, simply by
washing the treated lymphocyte preparations three to five
times with culture medium and then stimulating with PHA (7).
Thus, the suppressive factor appeared to bind relatively
weakly to a receptor on the lymphocyte surface, and to be
removed easily by washing. Using pharmacodynamic methods
analogous to a Lineweaver-Burke enzyme antagonism, we were
able to determine that PHA and the α-globulin factor bind to
separate receptors on the lymphocyte surface. The α-globulin
antagonism is a "non-competitive" type, i.e., antagonism that
does not involve alteration of the activation receptor.

These experiments further support the conclusion that the α-globulin inhibition occurs by altering a metabolic sequence that normally occurs subsequent to mitogen binding (7). A series of studies using the macrophage inhibition assay again supported this conclusion (9). When α-globulin fractions were added to an antigen sensitive population of peritoneal exudate cells, this factor prevented the macrophage immobilization that normally occurs upon exposure to antigen (Figure 3). When the system was separated, however, and macrophage immobilization was carried out by pre-exposure to MIF, the α-globulin failed to have any inhibitory effect. Thus, the α-globulin was further shown to have a selective effect upon early events involved in the immune response, and not to effect macrophage sensitization or migratory response to antigen.

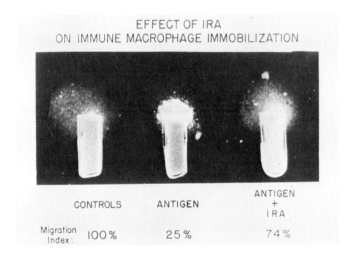

Figure 3. Effect of suppressor α-globulin (IRA) on macrophage migration. The inhibition of migration induced by antigen was reversed, as determined by planimetric measurement of the area of cellular out-growth.

As we began to appreciate the selective immunoinhibitory
activity of the serum factor, we started to think of it as
part of a natural immunoregulatory system -- a system which
at that time was not fully appreciated by the immunologic
community. We chose to label this serum factor
"Immunoregulatory Alpha-Globulin" or IRA (6).

We then performed a series of *in vivo* studies examining
the effect of the IRA on primary and secondary antibody synthesis (8,10,35). The plaque forming cell response to SRBC
was used as the assay system; the response was suppressed
with human α-globulin fractions. Human or bovine serum
albumin (and occasionally other non-suppressive α-globulin
fractions) was employed as control to examine for any effects
of foreign protein upon this assay system. We found that
administration of the IRA 24 hours prior to antigen resulted
in a marked suppression of the primary 19S plaque forming
cell response (Figure 4). Administration after antigen had
no effect. Using the inhibition of the primary plaque
forming cell response as an assay, we determined the
biological half-life of the human factor in mice (8). For
this experiment a series of mice were all given an 80% suppressive dose of IRA; then sequentially (every day) one
group of mice was given SRBC and the direct plaque forming
cell response measured four days later. Figure 5
demonstrates the progressive loss of suppressive activity
from these animals. There was a loss of 50% of suppressive
activity about four days following the IRA administration,
and a complete loss within eight days.

Although somewhat more complex, the α-globulin also had
an inhibitory effect upon the secondary antibody response
(10). When the factor was administered prior to primary
antigen exposure, both the direct and indirect secondary
plaque forming cell responses were reduced some 15 days later.
These animals acted as though they had been primed and produced
a rapid, but reduced plaque forming cell response upon
secondary challenge. When the IRA was administered 24 hours
prior to a secondary challenge with antigen, there was a
marked reduction in the secondary direct plaque forming cell
response, and much less inhibition of the indirect plaque ,
forming cell response; but even here a significant inhibition
was apparent. Control experiments demonstrated that the IRA
did not interfere with antibody secretion by plaque forming
cells. Using hemagglutinating antibody and a variety of

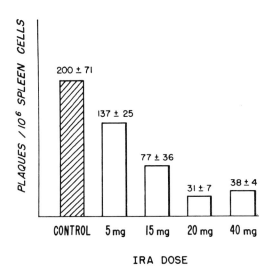

Figure 4. Dose dependent suppression by IRA of
antibody plaque forming cell response in
C57Bl/6J mice immunized with sheep erythrocytes
(SRBC). Protocol involved intravenous
administration of IRA 24 hours prior to antigen.
Direct plaque forming cell response determined
four days following SRBC. Control included
crystalline human serum albumin at 40 mg/ml.

different antigens (bound to indicator erythrocytes), we
demonstrated that the IRA did not interfere with antibody
binding to antigen. Thus, the IRA could antagonize both
primary and secondary antibody responses with a thymus
dependent antigen. When we examined the response of these
mice to a thymus independent antigen, *E. coli* lipopoly-
saccharide, the results were entirely different (11). Using
endotoxin 055:B5, we found we could <u>not</u> inhibit the plaque
forming cell response to this antigen. Thus, the IRA
appeared to have further specificity in its inhibitory
effect, acting selectively on T cells.

Studies on T and B cell rosette formation yielded data
further supporting our observations of the selective effects

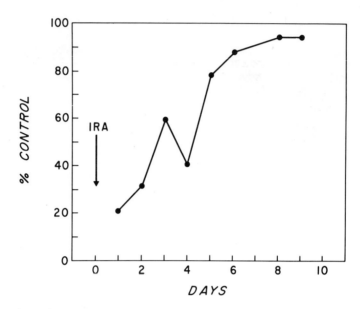

Figure 5. *In vivo* duration of suppressive effect
following one injection of an 80% suppressor
dose of α– globulin (IRA) (on day 0). Sheep
erythrocytes (SRBC) administered to groups of
C57B1/6J mice sequentially each day for nine
days. Plaque forming cell response determined
four days after administration of SRBC. Data
presented are compared to human serum albumin
control population, corrected to PFC/10^6
splenocytes.

of IRA. While studying the generation of SRBC-rosette
forming cells in mouse spleens, we performed a control experiment in which we incubated immune spleen cells with SRBC in
the presence of IRA. The splenocytes so treated failed to
produce normal numbers of rosettes. We subsequently
discovered that simply adding IRA would antagonize the
spontaneous rosettes formed between T lymphocytes and SRBC
using both murine spleen cells and human peripheral blood
lymphocytes. When we examined the effect of IRA upon the
rosette formation that occurs between complement-bearing

erythrocytes (EAC cells) and B cells (with receptors for C3b)
we found that the α-globulin did not antagonize this rosette
formation (a typical experiment is presented in Table I).
The antagonism of T-cell rosette formation is not in itself
unique. A variety of exogenous agents have been demonstrated
to produce the same kind of antagonism, including metabolic
antagonists that inhibit oxidative phosphorylation (13),
glycolysis (14), or microfilament function (15); also those
that antagonize protein and nucleic acid synthesis (16),
divalent cation movement across the plasma membrane (13), and
those that alter cyclic nucleotide levels (such as cholera
endotoxin) (17). Since the α-globulin does not appear to
have non-specific effects on cell metabolism, cell movement,
or protein and nucleic acid synthesis, it may be that its
mechanism of action involves the selective alteration, intra-
cellularly, of cyclic nucleotide concentrations in the T
cell. However, there are not yet sufficient data to draw any
such conclusion.

During the course of our investigations, we also
observed that immune lymphocyte populations incubated with
antigen in the presence of IRA failed to bind antigen, at
least in the same quantities as controls incubated with
albumin or whole serum (69,70). The phenomenon was first
observed using a variety of antigens bound to tanned carrier
erythrocytes and assayed as rosettes; there was approximately
50% reduction in immunocyte-rosettes in the presence of IRA.
The IRA did not alter antigen recognition by antibody, since
it did not interfere with antibody agglutination. This
antagonism of antigen binding by lymphocytes was confirmed in
subsequent experiments using soluble antigen in an equilibrium system. Preliminary data, using the equilibrium
methodology, suggest no decrease in antigen binding capacity,
but rather a reduction in antigen binding affinity. The
mechanism of action for this effect, and the exact cell
populations involved remain to be determined.

Studies carried out by other investigators have confirmed or extended some of our observations, and in some
cases, have produced conflicting results. Milton (21),
Yachnin (24), and others (19,23,25,30,37) have also demonstrated inhibition of mitogen induced lymphocyte activation
by similar α-globulin containing fractions. Inhibition of
macrophage inhibitory factor (MIF) production has been
confirmed by Hanna and colleagues in Israel (42).

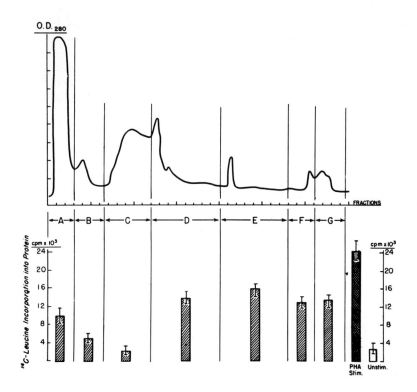

Figure 6. DEAE chromatographic separation of
immunosuppressive fractions from whole
plasma. Chromatography performed at pH 5.5
with an ascending linear salt gradient from
r/2 0.05 to r/2 0.5. Fractions were pooled
as noted (A,B,C, etc.), concentrations by
ultrafiltration on an Amicon UM 0.05 filter,
neutralized, dialyzed against tissue culture
media, sterilized by filtration through
Millipore 0.45 mμ filters and assayed for
suppression of PHA induced activation of human
blood lymphocyte cultures *in vitro.*

Mowbray (3), Glaser *et al.* (26), and others (18,27) have
observed the inhibition of a primary antibody response in
rabbits and mice with bovine and human fractions. A number
of investigators have confirmed the inhibition of graft
rejection in various animal systems (22,28). Glaser *et al.*
(26) and Nelken (32) have confirmed the ability of these

fractions to antagonize the spontaneous rosettes formed by
T cells with sheep erythrocytes. Conflicting observations
are reported by Glaser *et al.* (27), who found a more per-
manent inhibitory action of this factor on lymphocytes;
spleen cells from mice pretreated with IRA demonstrated
depressed immunity when adoptively administered to irradiated
isologous recipients. These authors also found that the IRA
had an inhibitory effect on the phagocytic activity of mouse
peritoneal macrophages towards *Staphylococcus albus*.

Nelken (32) has also observed an inhibition of antigen
binding with immune lymphocytes. Morse *et al.* (33) have
confirmed the selective anti-proliferative effect on T cells,
with no apparent effect on B cells. Milton and Mowbray (43)
observed the reversible loss of receptors for the mitogen
PHA and anti-immunoglobulin G antibody on lymphocyte
surfaces. These authors have consistently found that their
preparations demonstrate considerable RNAase activity, and
have suggested that the loss of receptors might result from
selective RNAase destruction of messenger RNA. They
hypothesize that the loss of surface receptors results from
a subsequent lack of mRNA directed new protein synthesis to
replace normal turnover. This would not appear to be the
mechanism of action involved in the peptide factor, since
these preparations do not contain any RNAase activity (*vide
infra*).

CHARACTERIZATION OF THE SERUM SUPPRESSOR

During the past seven years we have attempted to isolate
and purify the serum suppressor factor present among the α-
globulin proteins of normal plasma. This has proven to be a
difficult task. Initially, we obtained our active fractions
by chromatography of whole human plasma on DEAE cellulose at
pH 5.5 with a linear salt gradient from r/2 0.05 to 0.5
(Figure 6). About 80% of these plasma batches yielded one or
more suppressive fractions, generally in the third or fourth
peak eluted from the column. The factor(s) so isolated were
non-dialysable (at neutral pH's), heat stable at 56°C for
30 minutes, and non-sedimentable by ultracentrifugation at
100,000 X g for one hour. Ouchterlony analysis of active and

inactive fractions using a panel of antisera against the common α-globulins failed to demonstrate the consistent presence of any identifiable α-globulin protein in fractions with suppressive activity, or its absence in fractions without suppressive activity.

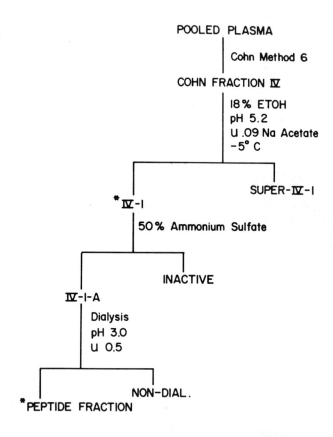

POOLED PLASMA

| Cohn Method 6

COHN FRACTION Ⅳ

18% ETOH
pH 5.2
U .09 Na Acetate
-5° C

SUPER-Ⅳ-I

*Ⅳ-I

50% Ammonium Sulfate

INACTIVE

Ⅳ-I-A

Dialysis
pH 3.0
U 0.5

NON-DIAL.

*PEPTIDE FRACTION

Figure 7. Fractionation scheme for the preparation of an immunosuppressive peptide fraction from immunosuppressor α-globulin protein precursor.

Using Cohn Method 6 to fractionate plasma (44), it was
subsequently found that Fraction IV, sometimes Fraction V,
and less often Fraction VI, contained the suppressive
activity. We therefore began to use large pools of frozen
Fraction IV as our starting material, obtained by the
Massachusetts State Biological Laboratories, during the preparation of albumin, and found that sub-fraction IV-1 of
Fraction IV could yield suppressive activity (31). We subsequently discovered that the suppressive activity was
precipitable with ammonium sulfate at 40-50% of saturation,
and thereafter used this procedure prior to DEAE chromatography (Figure 7). Under these conditions greater than 90%
of our isolation experiments yielded a suppressive fraction.
As we experimented with elution conditions, however, we began
to find suppressive activity in many different fractions.
This occurred especially when elution pH's were at pH 5 or
below. These observations suggested that the suppressive
activity might result from a small fragment of the α-globulin
which could be partially dissociated in acid buffers. Subsequent experiments demonstrated this to be the case (31).
We ultimately produced a dialysable fraction that appeared
to contain all the biological activity previously demonstrated in the non-dialysable precursor.

Biologically, the peptide fraction antagonizes graft
rejection (45) and antibody formation (12) and augments tumor
growth in murine animal models (46). It antagonizes lymphocyte activation *in vitro* and prevents T cell rosette formation (11,12). When injected into intact mice, the peptide
fraction is also shown to have a biologic half-life of four
days, the same as the macromolecular precursor. This
observation supports the notion that the factor is naturally
bound to an α-globulin carrier, and is not an artificial
cleavage product resulting from the isolation procedure.

We have not yet been able to remove all suppressive
activity by acid dialysis; moreover, we do not know if the
IRA peptide factor is the only suppressive factor, or if
there are additional factors. Recent experiments by Miller
(37) suggest, in fact, the presence of two factors with
dissimilar thermal sensitivity.

The peptide fraction has been further purified by high
voltage electrophoresis, but we still do not have a single

purified substance. The suppressive peptide fractions isolated thus far do not appear to contain a significant amount
of carbohydrate, nor are they labile to lipid (ether)
extraction. The biological activity is destroyed by trypsin
and chymotrypsin, and (more slowly) be pepsin. Almost all of
the weight of the material can be accounted for as peptide.
The apparent molecular weight of the active material.
estimated by ultracentrifugation and gel filtration, is
approximately 5,000 - 7,000 daltons.

Serum or plasma from patients with a number of unusual
clinical states has been found to contain immunosuppressive
substances different from those isolated from normal plasma.
Field and Caspary (50) and their associates found a "lymphocytes depressive factor" (LDF) in the serum of cancer
patients. The serum concentration of this substance
correlated with increasing mass of tumor. They later demonstrated that this factor could be isolated with a fraction
containing predominantly α_2-macroglobulin (36). However, a
much smaller peptide suppressor factor could be separated
from this macroglobulin fraction by reagents which reduce
disulfide bonds. Our laboratories have been able to isolate
an IRA-like peptide from the serum of a variety of cancer
patients (more detail about this will be presented below).
Recent reports by Hakoma et al. (40) and by Mortenson et al.
(41) have demonstrated that purified human C-reactive protein
(a protein appearing in the plasma in a variety of inflammatory states) preferentially binds to T lymphocytes, and
antagonizes T-cell rosette formation with sheep erythrocytes
using human and murine T cells, and prevents T-cell blast
response to PHA or to a mixed leukocyte culture. It has been
demonstrated by a number of investigators that fetal serum
(72) and serum from pregnant females (73-76,79,80) are mildly
immunosuppressive. Although the exact factor(s) responsible
for this phenomenon have not yet been separated, the recent
demonstration of suppressive activity by α-fetoprotein (39,
77) raises the possibility of its involvement in pregnancy-
related phenomena. Preliminary studies with antisera to
human α-fetoprotein do not demonstrate any precipitin
reactions between IRA containing protein or peptide fractions
(to a detectable level of 1 µg/ml).

A number of recent studies have suggested that interferon may have immunoinhibitory effects. Most of these

reports have utilized interferons produced *in vitro*, but interferon does appear as a humoral factor in the plasma under appropriate stimulation. Interferons have generally been found to antagonize proliferative events induced by mitogens (100,101) or in graft rejection (102,103). However, Chester *et al.* (104) using interferon in mouse serum, demonstrated an ability to antagonize antibody formation also. The dose required for this was 10-100 fold greater than that required to prevent lethal cytocidal virus infection. However, Thorbecke *et al.* (105) have suggested that the immunosuppressive effects of interferon are not specific for immunocytes and are similar to interferon effect on cell proliferation in general.

Most of the serum factors appear to have activity directed primarily against T lymphocytes. This is true for IRA and C-reactive protein, but not yet defined for α-fetoprotein. At least one patient with common variable (acquired) hypogammaglobulinemia has been reported (78) whose serum appears to contain a factor(s) with selective suppressor effects upon B cell activation. This serum contains a factor that antagonizes T cell derived mitogenic factor activation of B lymphocytes.

Until these individual factors found in clinical situations have been isolated, purified and analyzed by chemical and immunochemical methods in a number of laboratories, it is not possible to tell whether they are a variety of different substances having similar biological functions, or if they are only carriers for a common suppressor peptide. This is particularly difficult since it has been our experience that the IRA peptide suppressor may bind to a number of carrier macromolecules.

ORIGIN AND BIOLOGICAL SIGNIFICANCE
OF THE SERUM SUPPRESSOR FACTORS

The biological significance of serum immunosuppressive factors remains to be fully determined. The α-fetoprotein may play an important regulatory role in the maternal-fetal immuno-interrelationship, but this is by no means established. C-reactive protein appears to be an acute phase reactant, and may arise in the liver (47), although it is also thought to arise at the site of local inflammation from leukocytes (48). The origin of the other factors is not known, and until origin can be determined it will be difficult to evaluate any functional role. Unfortunately, this is also true for the serum IRA-peptide suppressor which our laboratories have been studying in normal plasma. Despite this lack of knowledge about the origin, there are a number of clinical and experimental reports which collectively begin to suggest that these factors do have a significant biological role.

There is a large number of studies demonstrating that unfractionated serum/plasma extracted from a variety of clinical disease entities, may suppress one or another assay of lymphocyte function *in vitro*. For example, suppressive factors have been suggested to be present in the serum of patients with tuberculosis (81), multiple sclerosis (82), chronic cutaneous candidiasis (83), hepatitis (51,84), rheumatoid arthritis (85), ataxia telangiectasia (49) and cancer (50,86-96). All of these diseases are associated with intense antigenic stimulation. Unfortunately many of these studies with whole serum suffer from an inability to distinguish a reduction in stimulatory co-factors (which interact with the bioassay system employed) from increased suppressor activity.

Several investigators have hypothesized that some relationship exists between immune responses and some of the proteins that migrate as α-globulins. Riggio *et al.* (19) were the first to suggest that the serum suppressor which is found in the serum α-globulins might become elevated during immune reactivity. These investigators found that serum α_2-globulin levels became elevated during rejection crises in patients undergoing human kidney transplants. They subsequently isolated an α-globulin fraction from such patients and demonstrated increased suppressive activity in these fractions. MacFarlin and Oppenheim (49) have also found a correlation of suppressor activity in serum and increased α-globulins in patients with ataxia telangiectasia. Field and Caspary (50) and Hsu and Logerfo (51) have carried out similar analyses in cancer bearing patients. Recent work in our laboratories (97,98) has demonstrated a marked increase in IRA-like peptides in the serum of a variety of patients with advanced cancer.

A few investigators have recently begun to use experimental manipulations in animal model systems and in humans to determine which factors influence serum suppressor activity. Normal mouse serum contains a factor which inhibits the proliferation of mouse lymphocytes (108). In mouse serum this effect can be measured without isolation or concentration of the factor as is necessary with human or bovine plasma. Ashikawa *et al.* (22) followed the concentration of serum α-globulins during tumor growth in mice, and found that they rose as the tumor grew. He subsequently isolated the α-globulin from tumor bearing and control mice, and demonstrated increased suppressor activity in this fraction. Veit and Michael (29,99) have examined the possibility that the serum suppressor might be part of a normal host response to any antigenic challenge. Using mice immunized with erythrocytes, they demonstrated that the suppressor activity of serum increased within 24 hours following antigenic administration and remained elevated for at least five days more. They also demonstrated that this suppressor activity resided in the α-globulins. Using adoptive transfer experiments into irradiated syngeneic recipients, they found that the serum suppressor seemed to be derived from a bone marrow cellular element activated shortly after antigenic exposure. In support of this concept is the study by Bullock and Möller (106) that suggests that murine lymphoid cells exist in a partially suppressed state *in vivo*, and that this suppression may be easily removed by washing the cells and establishing them in a milieu containing fetal calf serum. Burger *et al.* (52,109) have extended this idea to cell mediated immunity. They have followed the concentration of serum α-globulin during the development of delayed hypersensitivity in the guinea pig, and have demonstrated a reduction in skin hypersensitivity at the same time that the serum α-globulins increase.

Some recent experiments by Benson *et al.* (107) suggest that the serum suppressor factor in murine serum may be related to the formation of amyloidosis. These investigators found that there is a marked increase in α-globulins, and suppressor activity of mice during the development of casein-induced amyloid; using an antisera to the AA protein fraction of amyloid fibrils they found they could selectively block the serum suppressive activity in both amyloid forming mice, and also in normal mouse serum.

Unfortunately, most of the studies cited above cannot determine if the suppressive activity they are measuring is the same factor present in normal plasma, or if new factors are added by the clinical or experimental state.

A real understanding of the natural role played by these serum suppressive factors must await better assay methods, specific for each material, as well as a clearer under-standing of their origin. This phase of the research is only just beginning with α-fetoprotein and C-reactive protein, and is not yet possible with the other factors. However, a picture of increased serum suppression occurring along with stimulation or antagonism of immunity is beginning to emerge. This is further supported by the increasing numbers of reports of immunosuppressive factors isolated from sources other than plasma or serum.

NATURAL SUPPRESSORS FROM SOURCES OTHER THAN SERUM OR PLASMA

Factors which suppress one or more aspects of immunity have been extracted or isolated from various tissues. Not all of these substances have been examined critically for the cell specificity of their inhibitory functions, and many have only been assayed by inhibition of ^{3}H-thymidine incorporation into DNA by lymphocytes. Thus, it becomes difficult to tell whether some of the factors reported below represent true immunosuppressive materials, or merely cytostatic agents and/or substances which alter the uptake of radioactive precursors. Despite these difficulties, a picture begins to emerge of immunosuppressive materials present in many tissues and cells involved in immune reactivity, influencing different parts of the immune response.

Thymus and Bursa of Fabricius.

The thymus contains substances antagonistic to

lymphocyte activation. Carpenter and colleagues (53-55) have extracted a macromolecular substance from bovine thymus glands that is immunosuppressive both *in vivo* and *in vitro*. Their extraction and purification procedures are similar to those described by Mowbray (2,3) for the isolation of serum factors. The factor thus isolated has many similarities to the serum factor, but differs in its failure to antagonize MIF production, lymphocyte mediated toxicity, and rosettes. It is also five to ten times more active per unit weight than the most pure of the serum factors currently available. Kiger *et al.* (56-58) in Paris, have extracted a water soluble factor which is not precipitable with 42% ethanol, and which antagonizes PHA-induced stimulation of DNA synthesis in blood lymphocyte cultures. Their factor was estimated to have a molecular weight of about 20,000 daltons by gel filtration. No such factor was able to be isolated from kidney controls using the same methodology. This factor was also found to antagonize antibody formation and graft vs host reaction in mice *in vivo*. In 1969 (59), our laboratory observed the production of a factor that antagonized lymphocyte proliferation produced by cultures of human thymic stroma. We did not determine, however, whether this factor was immunosuppressive *in vivo* and have not characterized it further. Danielson and Van Alten (117) have extracted a suppressor factor from chicken Bursa of Fabricius.

Peripheral Lymphoid Tissues.

A number of investigators have extracted immunosuppressive substances from lymph nodes or spleens. Moorhead *et al.* (60), in 1969, were the first to demonstrate that a water extract of porcine lymph nodes could antagonize PHA-induced mitosis and DNA synthesis of blood lymphocyte cultures without apparent cytotoxicity. Garcia-Firalt and coworkers (61-63) have repeated these experiments with calf tissue (and peripheral blood lymphocytes), separating a 45,000 dalton molecular weight inhibitor by precipitation with 75% ethanol. Houck *et al.* (64,65) confirmed and extended these observations by demonstrating that similar extracts from calf spleen and thymus could inhibit MIF production by human blood lymphocytes *in vitro*. In recent years these extracted factors have been named "chalones" (66) and are assumed to function as part of a regulatory mechanism maintaining the size of lymphoid tissues.

Lymphoid Cells.

Ambrose (67) was the first to demonstrate that antigen stimulated cultures of rabbit lymphoid cells could produce a protein factor capable of inhibiting a secondary antibody response when transferred to other cell cultures responding to a second antigen. Since that time a number of investigators have observed suppressive factors produced by lymphoid cells from one or another source. Antigen stimulation of normal murine spleen cells in culture cause the production of suppressor substances which antagonize antibody response to an unrelated antigen when passed to syngeneic cells *in vitro* (111-117). Rich and Pierce (116) have studied in more detail the production of one such inhibitory factor induced by mitogenic (Con A) stimulation of murine spleen cells. They found their factor antagonized only the early events involved in immune response to antigen, and had no effect when added to lymphocytes 48 hours or more after antigen exposure. Recent experiments suggest that the macrophage population is the target of this effector substance.

A number of investigators have observed the production of suppressor substances by lymphocyte cell lines in tissue culture. Smith and coworkers (68) have demonstrated that some lymphoblast lines produce an "inhibitor of DNA synthesis" (IDS) that acts to inhibit DNA synthesis in normal blood lymphocyte cultures. Their factor appeared to act only at the time of activation of lymphocyte stimulation and had little effect when added 24 hours after the activation of blood cells. The effect was reversible with washing. Unfortunately, their factor also inhibited DNA synthesis in L cell cultures, but upon morphological examination, did not appear to antagonize blast transformation. These authors later suggested that the factor was most likely related to mycoplasma contamination of the lymphoblast line. However, other investigators have observed several phenomena which do not appear to be related to mycoplasma contamination. Hersh *et al.* (71) reported the production of a proteinaceous factor by human lymphoma cells which selectively antagonized other lymphocyte activation, measured by DNA synthesis or blast transformation. This factor was found to be lymphocyte specific and also species specific in its activity. Takado *et al.* (110) have observed a factor produced by the MOLT cell line which antagonizes antibody formation. Green *et al.* (118 119) have demonstrated the production of a factor which antagonizes mitogenic stimulation of normal blast lymphocytes. Their factor is produced under conditions which create crowding in the lymphoblast cultures.

It should be emphasized that the production of suppressive factors by various lymphoid cell cultures is by no means a simple and clearly understood phenomenon. A number of investigators have reported the production of "stimulatory" substances under circumstances which sometimes yield suppressive materials (120-123), but generally from cultures containing predominantly T cells. Although the subject of stimulatory factors is beyond the scope of this review, it is important to realize that a number of investigators (111-115, 126) have been able to find both stimulatory and/or suppressive activity (not related to a specific antigen) in the same supernate obtained from appropriately stimulated cells. The expression of one or the other of these factors was dependent upon technical details of the assay systems employed in measuring them, e.g., time of administration in relation to antigen; concentration of factor; numbers of responding cells, etc. It is not clear from currently available data if these different and antagonistic actions reflect mixtures of different factors or if one factor may have multiple actions depending upon the time and manner of presentation to its target cell population.

Macrophages.

At least four laboratories (125-128) have reported the production of humoral factors by macrophage cultures (or at least adherent peritoneal exudate cells), that antagonize lymphocyte activation measured by DNA synthesis or protein synthesis from radioactive precursors. These observations succeed a number of studies demonstrating that macrophages may have inhibitory effects upon immune responses when added to responding lymphocytes *in vitro* (129-132). Waldman and Gottlieb (125) and Calderon *et al.* (127) have characterized their factors as dialysable and heat stable to 70°C. Nelson (126) has found that macrophages from mice need to be "activated" by one or another endotoxins before this factor is produced. It is unclear if this suppressive effect is limited to immune responses. Calderon *et al.* (128) have observed that this factor antagonizes the incorporation of ^{3}H-thymidine into DNA by a variety of cells other than lymphocytes. Opitz *et al.* (128) suggest that the factor may influence the metabolic use of radioactive thymidine by lymphocytes (and other cells), and is not necessarily an inhibitor of lymphocyte proliferation. Further work on this macrophage factor must be carried out before the full biological significance of the material is appreciated.

Plasma Cells.

It is a well known phenomenon that patients and animals bearing plasma cell tumors have a reduced capacity to produce normal antibodies with minimal loss of cellular immunity (133,134). Zolla and coworkers (134) were the first to suggest that this phenomenon could result from a humoral factor released by the plasma cell tumors. They have recently shown that such a humoral factor exists (135), which has a selective inhibitory effect upon B cells with minimal or no effect on T cell function. It remains to be determined if the inhibitory factor observed under these experimental conditions with tumors reflects a physiological control mechanism that normally occurs in B cell maturation (but is even more easily observed because of the large numbers of plasma cells available in the tumor), or if this is an abnormal mechanism that occurs only under tumor circumstances. For purposes of this review, we have assumed that these observations reflect a regulatory mechanism involved in B cell maturation, because the investigators have demonstrated that the production of this factor is unique to plasmacytomas and is not associated with other lymphoid or nonlymphoid tumors, and because a factor in serum with similar properties has been observed (78).

Placenta and Amniotic Fluid.

In 1971, Riggio *et al.* demonstrated that the placenta contains a glycoprotein factor capable of antagonizing human lymphocyte activation by mitogens. This factor was extractable with 0.6 N perchloric acid, and was subsequently separated by DEAE chromatography. It appeared to be a nondialysable protein with α-globulin-like (pre- and post-albumin) characteristics. In 1973 St. Hill *et al.* (73)

suggested that pregnant and fetal serum were immunosuppressive, and in 1974 Belanger *et al.* (77) suggested that this
might result from the presence of α-fetoprotein in these
fluids. At the same time, Ogra *et al.* (137) demonstrated
that amniotic fluid could antagonize antibody responses to
sheep erythrocytes in a primary antibody response *in vitro*.
They subsequently extracted the protein responsible for this
inhibitory effect and demonstrated that it was α-fetoprotein (39).

Liver.

A lymphocyte inhibitory factor has also been isolated
from the cytoplasm of normal human liver using gel filtration
(138). This factor inhibited ^{3}H-thymidine uptake by mitogen
stimulated blood lymphocytes, but not by HeLa cell.

Cancer.

There is an increasing amount of data supporting the
notion that cancer cells may produce, or cause other cells to
produce, humoral immunosuppressive factors. A comprehensive
review of this literature is beyond the scope of this manuscript, but humoral immunosuppressive factors have been
observed in the serum of cancer patients (22,50,92,94-97,139-
141), in the ascites bathing cancer cells 142-150), and in
the medium bathing tumor cell culture (151-153), and as
extracts directly derived from tumor or cells (154,155). How
these various substances act, how they are produced, and upon
which cell populations of the immune response they act, are
still unanswered questions. It is not clear whether these
substances are similar or dissimilar molecules. The cancer
bearing patient is frequently immunosuppressed, and
sufficient data are accumulated to support the hypothesis
that this state may result in part, from humoral immunoinhibitory factors produced or induced by the cancer.

SUMMARY

In summary, there exists a large number of natural immunosuppressive factors that may be found in serum, lymphoid tissues, and non-lymphoid tissues such as liver, placenta, amniotic fluid, and in cancer tissue. How many of the different factors are identical or represent differences which are apparent only because of the assay systems used to measure them, is impossible to tell. Most such factors have not yet been well characterized, but those that have been partially purified appear to be either macromolecular proteins or peptides. These factors may act upon different cell populations of the immune response, but most have been assayed using T lymphocyte dependent systems. However, some factors have been described that appear to have selective effects on either B cells or macrophages.

The true biological significance of these diverse factors remains to be determined. Progress in this area of under-standing, however, will probably be dependent upon selective immunochemical assays rather than the contemporary bioassays used to observe and define these factors. Most bioassays are too crude and contain too many antagonistic and dependent variables or modifying compounds to permit accurate quantita-tive measurement of changes occurring within any single factor during immune reactivity.

ACKNOWLEDGEMENTS

This work was supported in part by Research Grants CA-15129, CA 15848 and AM 10824 from the United States Public Health Service and Army Contract DA 49-193-MD-2621.

Table I

Human Lymphocyte "T" and "B" Rosettes[*]

	Rosettes/10^3 Lymphocytes[†]	% Suppression
Control	272 ± 25.8	----
NHS 4 mg/ml	250 ± 20.4	0
IRA 4 mg/ml	17 ± 12.5	93.7
EAC Rosettes	80 ± 10.3	----
NHS 4 mg/ml	83 ± 6.4	0
IRA 4 mg/ml	81 ± 8.5	0

[*] *Effect of immunosuppressive α-globulin (IRA) on T and B cell rosette formation with human blood lymphocytes. T cell rosettes formed with sheep erythrocytes after sedimentation and incubation at 4°C for ten minutes. IRA or control human serum albumin added 30 minutes prior to addition of SRBC. B cell rosettes formed with antibody and human complement coated erythrocytes (EAC) at 4°C for ten minutes. As above, IRA and HSA were added 30 minutes prior to EAC cells.*

[†] *Mean and S.D. or 4 determinations.*

Table II

Isolation of Suppressor

Reference Number	Source of α-Globulin	Fractionation Method	Dose Range	Assay	
				Species	
(1)	rat human	Cohn Fraction.IV	18-30 mg	rat	
(2)	bovine human rabbit	DEAE Chromatog.	100 mg	rabbit	
(3)	rat rabbit human bovine	DEAE Chromatog.	25-100 mg	rat rabbit	
(4)	human	DEAE Chromatog.	100 mg 5 mg	rabbit rat	
(18)	bovine	DEAE Chromatog.	12.5 mg	mice	
(5)	human	DEAE Chromatog.	1-4 mg/ml	human cells in culture	

Table II

Factors From Serum

Assay System	Results
in vivo skin allograft	41.5% survival to 60 days
in vivo hemagglutinin and precipitation titre	80% inhibition of control; time dependent
in vivo skin allograft	35% survival for 30 days, 20% survival for 8 months
in vivo skin allograft	rabbit-up to 33 days survival rat-up to 20 days survival
in vivo primary antibody response to SRBC	decreased antibody titer, $\log_2$, 0.77
in vitro lymphocyte response to mitogens and antigens	90% inhibition of protein and DNA synthesis, 90% blast transformation

Table II (contd)

Reference Number	Source of α-Globulin	Fractionation Method	Dose Range	Assay Species
(20)	human	not specified	3^x 150-200 µg	rabbit
(19)	human	0.4 N HClO$_4$ solubil., DEAE Chromatog. 0.12 M	0.5-1.5 mg/ml	human cells in culture
(6)	human	DEAE Chromatog. Fraction IV	0.2-4.0 mg/ml	human cells in culture
(8)	human	DEAE Chromatog. Fraction IV	5-40 mg	mice
(21)	bovine	DEAE Chromatog. Fraction C	0.05-0.20 mg/ml	human cells in culture
(10)	human	DEAE Chromatog. Fraction IV	20 mg	mice
(22)	human cancer murine	Prep. electrophoresis α-globulins	3 x 115 mg	mice

Table II (contd)

Assay System	Results
in vivo anti-bacterial antibody titre	90% suppression of production of circulating antibodies, time dose dependent
in vitro lymphocyte response to PHA	89% inhibition of ^{3}H-thymidine uptake
in vitro lymphocyte response to PHA	77% suppression of protein synthesis
in vivo antibody plaque forming cell response	graded inhibition of primary PFC at doses between 5-20 mg/mouse, 80% maximum inhibition
mixed lymphocyte response to antigens or mitogens	80% inhibition of DNA synthesis at optimal dose
in vivo PFC response	7/10 experiments yielded 80% suppression of secondary antibody response
in vivo skin homografts and GVH (Simonsen's assay)	prolongation of grafts from 10.2-19.3 days, 50% reduction in GVH

Table II (contd)

Reference Number	Source of α-Globulin	Fractionation Method	Dose Range	Assay Species
(23)	human cancer	Sephadex G-200 Peak IV (peptide)	unspecified	human cells in culture
(38)	human	Heat stable (100°C) peptide from Cohn IV	0.05-1.0 mg/ml	human cells in culture
(9)	human guniea pig	DEAE Chromatog. Fraction IV	1-4 mg/ml	guinea pig peritoneal cells in culture
(24)	human	DEAE Chromatog.	1-4 mg/ml	human cells in culture
(25)	human cancer & preg.	unspecified, M.W. 520,000 α-globulin	unspecified	human cells in culture
(26)	human	DEAE Chromatog. Peak 3-4	1-6 mg/ml	rat

Table II (contd)

Assay System	Results
in vivo DNA synthesis induced by antigen (PPD)	80-90% inhibition of antigen-induced DNA synthesis
in vitro lymphocyte response to PHA	suppression with heat stable peptide higher specific activity than starting protein
in vitro macrophage immobilization	80% inhibition of antigen-induced immobilization
in vitro lymphocyte response to antigens and mitogens	dose dependent inhibition of suppression (between 2-3 mg/ml)
in vitro mixed leukocyte culture reactivity	inhibition of ^{3}H-thymidine uptake
in vivo hemolytic PFC and antigen rosette formation	90% inhibition RFC, 85% inhibition of primary and secondary PFC response at 3 mg/ml

Table II (contd)

Reference Number	Source of α-Globulin	Fractionation Method	Dose Range	Assay Species
(27)	human	DEAE Chromatog. Peak 3-4	20 mg/ml	rat mouse
(28)	human	DEAE Chromatog. Peak 3-4	20 mg	rat
(7)	human	DEAE Chromatog. Cohn, Fraction IV Peak 3	2-4 mg/ml	human cells in culture
(43)	bovine	DEAE Chromatog.		mouse rat human
(29)	mouse	NH_4SO_4 precip. & G 200 gel filtration	0.1-1.0 mg/ml	mouse splenocytes in culture

Table II (contd)

Assay System	Results
in vivo hemagglutinin titre, *in vitro* effect on phagocytic cell bacteria killing	suppression of 1^{ary} and 2^{ary} response to SRBC; reduction in phagocytic killing of bacteria; inability of splenocytes from treated mice to restore immune response
in vivo skin allograft	prolongation of graft survival from 9.2 to 17.7 days; additive effects with cortisol and ALS
in vitro lymphocyte response to mitogens and antigens	inhibition of lymphocyte proliferation. Temporal studies, receptor studies -- reversibility
PHA binding Ant. IgG binding PPD stimulation	reversible loss of receptors for PHA and anti-IgG. Reversible inhibition of PPD stimulation; suggest due to RNAase destruction of mRNA
in vitro Mishell Dutton primary antibody response to SRBC	soluble in 60% NH_4SO_4, macroglobulin on gel filtration; sharp dose/time response curves

Table II (contd)

Reference Number	Source of α-globulin	Fractionation Method	Dose Range	Assay Species
(30)	bovine	DEAE Chromatog. 0.2-0.5 M peak	0.1-2.0 mg/ml	bovine blood cells in culture
(31)	human	Cohn Fraction. NH_4SO_4 solubil., peptide produced by acid dialysis	0.2-4 mg/ml	human cells in culture, mouse
(32)	ACD Blood	DEAE Chromatog. 0.2 M peak	2-4.5 mg	mouse
(33)	human	DEAE Chromatog.	0.25-4 mg/ml	human cells in culture
(11)	human	Cohn IV, DEAE Chromatog.	15-40 mg	mouse
(34)	bovine	Sephadex G-200, peak III (albumin) boil for 9 min. ultra-filtration with Amicon filter	0.5 ml	mouse

Table II (contd)

Assay System	Results
in vitro lymphocyte DNA synthesis stimulated by PPD and PHA	70% suppression of ^{3}H-thymidine uptake
in vitro lymphocyte response to mitogens and antigens; *in vivo* PFC primary response to SRBC (mice)	Cohn Fraction IV-1, precipitated by 50% NH_4SO_4; acid pH dependent release by dialysable peptide
in vivo allografts and xenografts	5.5-17 day survival of xenografts; 14.7-47 day survival of allografts
in vitro lymphocyte response to T and B mitogens	IRA suppresses T cells, no effect on B cell stimulators
in vivo PFC response to thymus dependent (SRBC) and independent antigens (endotoxin LPS)	thymus dependent antibody PFC 84.5% at 20 mg dose; no PFC suppression of LPS
in vivo PFC response to SRBC	factor is low MW, 8400 daltons heat stable

Table II (contd)

Reference Number	Source of α-Globulin	Fractionation Method	Dose Range	Assay Species
(35)	human	Cohn IV, DEAE Chromatog., protein; acid dialysis of above yielded peptide	15–30 mg; 1–5 mg peptide	mouse
(36)	human	G-200 gel filtration-α2-macroglobulin, protease sensitive, also derived peptide	50–150 μg/ml	human lymphocytes; guinea pig macrophage
(12)	human	Cohn IV, DEAE chromatog., acid dialysate peptide	6 mg peptide 20 mg protein *in vivo* 4 mg/ml human *in vitro*	mouse mouse human cells in culture
(37)	human	DEAE chromatog.	1–4 mg/ml	human, rabbit cells in culture
	rabbit	NH$_4$SO$_4$ precip.	1–4 mg/ml	mice
	bovine	G 200 gel filtration	1–4 mg/ml	guinea pig

Table II (contd)

Assay System	Results
in vivo PFC response to SRBC	80% suppression only when given prior to antigen
in vitro antigen stim. lymphocytes--supernatant assayed for macrophage slowing factor	α_2-macroglobulin demonstrates most activity (peptide separable with s-s reduction)
in vivo PFC response to SRBC and E. coli LPS *in vitro* - rosette formation SRBC and AEC human rosette assay	85% inhibition to SRBC Insignificant inhibition to E. coli LPS, 93% inhibition of rosette formation with SRBC, no inhibition of rosettes with EAC
in vitro responses to PHA ^{3}HT - DNA *in vivo* - Hemagglutination and PFC (primary response to SRBC) *in vivo* delayed hypersensitivity to DNCB	2 suppressor substances with different thermal sensitivity, 10-25,000 molecular weight & 60-70,000 molecular weight

Table II (contd)

Reference Number	Source of α-Globulin	Fractionation Method	Dose Range	Assay Species
(39)	murine	α-fetoprotein isolated by affinity chromatog. with antibody	1-200 µg/ml	mice
(40)	human (β-γ-globulin)	C-reactive protein precipitated with C-polysaccharide	4-75 µg/ml	human blood cells in culture
(41)	human (β-γ-globulin)	C-reactive protein isolated by affinity chromatog. with C-polysaccharide	25-200 µg/ml	human blood lym. " " murine splenic T cells

Table II (contd)

Assay System	Results
in vitro primary and secondary antibody response to SRBC	marked suppression by α-feto-protein in first 24 hours after antigen; not suppressive after 48 hours
in vitro-lymphocyte response to mitogen	inhibition of PHA, stimulation of ^{3}HT incorporation
fluorescent binding; mixed lymphocyte reaction; T cell rosettes w/SRBC; fluorescent binding	C-reactive protein binds selectively to T lymphocytes inhibits MLR as measured by ^{3}HT into DNA, inhibits T cell rosette formation

REFERENCES

1. Kamrin, B.B., Proc. Soc. Exp. Biol. Med., *100:* 58, 1959.

2. Mowbray, J.F., Transplantation, *1:* 15, 1963.

3. Mowbray, J.F., Immunology, *6:* 217, 1963.

4. Mannick, J.A. and Schmid, K., Transplantation, *5:* 1231, 1967.

5. Cooperband, S.R., Bondevik, H., Schmid, K. and Mannick, J.A., Science, *159:* 1243, 1968.

6. Cooperband, S.R., Davis, R.C., Schmid, K. and Mannick, J.A., Trans. Proc., *1:* 516, 1969.

7. Cooperband, S.R., Badger, A.M., Davis, R.C., Schmid, K. and Mannick, J.A., J. Immunol., *109:* 154, 1972.

8. Glasgow, A.H., Cooperband, S.R., Occhino, J.C., Schmid, K. and Mannick, J.A., Proc. Soc. Exp. Biol. Med., *138:* 753, 1971.

9. Davis, R.C., Cooperband, S.R. and Mannick, J.A., J. Immunol., *106:* 755, 1971.

10. Glasgow, A.H., Cooperband, S.R., Schmid, K., Parker, J.T. Occhino, J.C. and Mannick, J.A., Trans. Proc., *3:* 835, 1971.

11. Menzoian, J.O., Glasgow, A., Cooperband, S., Schmid, K., Saporoschetz, I. and Mannick, J.A., Trans. Proc., *5;* 141, 1973.

12. Menzoian, J.O., Glasgow, A.H., Nimberg, R.D., Cooperband, S.R., Schmid, K., Saporoschetz, I. and Mannick, J.A., J. Immunol., *113:* 266, 1974.

13. Bentwich, Z., Douglas, S.D., Siegal, F.D., Kunkel, H.G., Clin. Immunol. Immunopathol., *1:* 511, 1973.

14. Jondal, M., Holm, G., Wigzell, H., J. Exp. Med.,
    136: 207, 1972.

15. Kersey, J.H., Ham, D.J. and Buttrick, P., J. Immunol.,
    112: 862, 1974.

16. Bushkin, S.C., Pantic, V.S. and Incefy, G.S., Fed.
    Proc., *33*: 629, 1974.

17. Chisari, F.V. and Edgington, T.S., J. Exp. Med., *140*:
    1122, 1974.

18. Pullar, D.M., James, K. and Naysmith, J.D., Clin. Exp.
    Immunol., *3*: 457, 1968.

19. Riggio, R.R., Schwartz, G.H., Bull, F.G., Stenzel, K.H.,
    and Rubin, A.L., Transplantation, *8*: 689, 1969.

20. Whang, H.Y., Chun, D. and Neter, E., J. Immunol.,
    103: 824, 1969.

21. Milton, J.D., Immunology, *20*: 205, 1971.

22. Ashikawa, K., Inoue, K., Shimizu, T. and Ishibashi, Y.,
    Japan J. Exp. Med., *41*: 339, 1971.

23. Scheurlen, P.G., Schneider, W., Pappas, A., Lancet,
    2: 1265, 1971.

24. Yachnin, S., J. Immunol., *108*: 845, 1972.

25. Stimson, W.H., Lancet, *1*: 684, 1972.

26. Glaser, M., Cohen, I. and Nelken, D., J. Immunol.,
    108: 286, 1972.

27. Glaser, M., Ofek, I. and Nelken, D., Immunology, *23*: 205,
    1972.

28. Nelken, D. and Glaser, M., Proc. Soc. Exp. Biol. Med.,
    140: 996, 1972.

29. Veit, B. and Michael, G., J. Immunol., *111*: 341, 1973.

30. Outteridge, P.M. and Lepper, A.W.D., Immunology, *25*: 981,
    1973.

31. Occhino, J.C., Glasgow, A.H., Cooperband, S.R., Mannick, J.A. and Schmid, K., J. Immunol., *110*: 685, 1973.

32. Nelken, D., J. Immunol., *110*: 1161, 1973.

33. Morse, J.H., Morris, A.M. and Mascitelli, R., J. Clin. Invest., *52*: Abstract #212, 1973.

34. Karpas, A.B. and Segre, D., Proc. Soc. Exp. Biol. Med., *144*: 141, 1973.

35. Glasgow, A.H., Menzoian, J.O., Cooperband, S.R., Nimberg, R.D., Schmid, K. and Mannick, J.A., J. Immunol., *111*: 272, 1973.

36. Ford, W.H., Caspary, E.A. and Shenton, B., Clin. Exp. Immunol., *15*: 169, 1973.

37. Miller, F., Transplantation, in press, 1975.

38. Glasgow, A.H., Cooperband, S.R., Occhino, J.C., Schmid, K. and Mannick, J.A., Fed. Proc., *30*: 652, 1971.

39. Murgita, R.A. and Tomasi, T.B. Jr., J. Exp. Med., *141*: 269, 1975.

40. Hokama, Y., Pik, Y.P., Yanagihara, E. and Kimura, L., J. Ret. Soc., *13*: 111, 1973.

41. Mortenson, P.F., Osmand, A.P. and Gewurz, H., J. Exp. Med., *141*: 121, 1975.

42. Cooperband, S.R., Alpha-Globulins Affecting the Immune Response. Report of Immunology Workshop, in, *Progress in Immunology* II, Vol. 5, Edited by L. Brent and J. Holborow, p. 383-389, North-Holland Publishing Company, 1974; with particular reference to statement by Hanna, p. 384.

43. Milton, J.D. and Mowbray, J.F., Immunology, *23*: 599, 1972.

44. Cohn, E.J., Strong, L.E., Hughes, W.L., Mulford, D.J., Ashworth, J.M., Melin, M., Taylor, H.L., J. Am. Chem. Soc., *68*: 459, 1946.

45. Menzoian, J.O., Glasgow, A.H., Nimberg, R.B.,
    Constantian, M.B., Stevens, R.L., Cooperband, S.R.,
    Schmid, K. and Mannick, J.A., Transplantation, *18*: 391,'74

46. Glasgow, A.H., Cooperband, S.R. and Mannick, J.A.,
    Surgical Forum, *25*: 119, 1974.

47. Uete, T., Ogik, S., Fukaza, S. and Takuchi, Y., Clin.
    Biochem., *4*: 9, 1971.

48. Gay, S. and Geiler, G., Zeit. Ges. Imm. Med., *26*: 217,
    1971.

49. McFarlin, D.E. and Oppenheim, J.J., J. Immunol., *103*:
    1212, 1969.

50. Field, E.J. and Caspary, E.A., Brit. J. Cancer, *26*: 164,
    1972.

51. Hsu, C.C.S. and LoGerfo, P., Proc. Soc. Exp. Biol. Med.,
    139: 575, 1972.

52. Burger, D.R., Lilley, D.P., Reid, M., Irish, L., and
    Vetto, R.M., Cell. Immunol., *8*: 147, 1973.

53. Carpenter, C.B., in *Proceedings of the 4th Annual
    Leukocyte Culture Conference,* Edited by O.R. McIntyre,
    p. 317, Appleton-Century Crofts, Meredith Corp.,
    New York, 1971.

54. Carpenter, C.B., Boylston, A.W. II, and Merrill, J.P.,
    Cell. Immunol., *2*: 425, 1971.

55. Carpenter, C.B., Phillips, S.M. and Merrill, J.P., Cell.
    Immunol., *2*: 435, 1971.

56. Kiger, N., Florentin, I., Garcia-Giralt, E. and
    Mathe, G., Transp. Proc., *4*: 531, 1972.

57. Kiger, N., Europ. J. Clin. Biol. Res., *16*: 566, 1971.

58. Kiger, N., Florentin, I. and Methe, G., Transplantation,
    14: 448, 1972.

59. Davis, R.C., Cooperband, S.R. and Mannick, J.A., Surg.
    Forum, *20*: 244, 1969.

60. Moorhead, J.F., Paraskova-Tchernozenska, E., Pirrie, A.J. and Hayes, C., Nature, *224*: 1207, 1969.

61. Garcia-Giralt, E., LaSalvia, E., Florentin, I. and Mathe, G., Europ. J. Clin. Biol. Res., *15*: 1012, 1970.

62. LaSalvia, E., Garcia-Giralt, E., Macierira-Cuelho, A., Europ. J. Clin. Biol. Res., *15*: 789, 1970.

63. Morales, V.H. and Garcia-Giralt, E., Naturforschrift, *26*: 1139, 1971.

64. Houck, J.C., Irausquin, H. and Leikin, S., Science, *173*: 1139, 1971.

65. Houck, J.C., Attallah, A.M. and Lilly, J.R., Nature, *245*: 148, 1973.

66. Bullough, W.S., Biol. Review, *37*: 307, 1962.

67. Ambrose, C.T., J. Exp. Med., *130*: 1003, 1969.

68. Smith, R.T., Bauscher, J.A.C. and Adler, W.H., Am. J. Path., *60*: 495, 1970.

69. Glasgow, A.H., Cooperband, S.R. and Mannick, J.A., Fed. Proc., *31*: 803, 1972.

70. Glasgow, A.H., Cooperband, S.R., Schmid, K. and Mannick, J.A., J. Clin. Invest., *51*: 36a, 1972.

71. Hersh, E.M. and Drewinko, B., Cancer Res., *34*: 215, 1974.

72. Ayoub, J. and Kasakura, S., Clin. Exp. Immunol., *8*: 427, 1971.

73. St. Hill, C.A., Finn, R., Denye, V., Brit. Med. J., *5*: 513, 1973.

74. Curzon, P., Jones, E. and Gaugas, J., Brit. Med. J., *4*: 49, 1972.

75. Walker, J.S., Freeman, C.B. and Harris, R., Brit. Med. J. *3*: 469, 1972.

76. Leikin, S., Lancet, *2*: 43, 1972.

77. Belanger, L., Waithe, W., Daguillard, F.,
    Larochelle, J. and Dofour, D., in, *Proceedings of the*
    International Symposium on α-Fetoprotein, p. 423,
    St. Paul de Vence, France, 1974.

78. Gaha, R.S., Schneeberger, E., Merler, E. and Rosen, E.S.
    New Eng. J. Med., *291*: 1, 1974.

79. Kasakura, S., J. Immunol., *107*: 1296, 1971.

80. Buckley, R.H., Schiff, R.I. and Amos, D.A., J. Immunol.,
    108: 34, 1972.

81. Heilman, D.H. and MacFarland, W., Int. Arch. Allergy,
    30: 58, 1966.

82. Knowles, M., Hughes, D., Caspary, E.A. and Field, E.J.,
    Lancet, *2*: 1207, 1968.

83. Canales, L., Middlemas, R.O., Louro, J.M. and South, M.A.
    Lancet, *2*: 567, 1969.

84. Paronetto, F. and Popper, H., New Eng. J. Med., *283*: 277,
    1970.

85. McLaurin, B.D., Lancet, *1*: 1070, 1971.

86. Whittaker, M.G., Rees, K., and Clark, C.G., Lancet,
    1: 892, 1971.

87. Garrioch, D.B., Good, R.A., and Gatti, R.A., Lancet,
    1: 618, 1970.

88. Gatti, R.A., Garrioch, D.B. and Good, R.A., in,
    Proceedings of Fifth Leukocyte Culture Conference,
    Edited by J. Harris, p. 339, New York, 1970.

89. Ricci, M., Passaleva, A. and Ricca, M., Lancet, *2*: 503,
    1966.

90. Sutherland, R.M., Inch, W.R. and McCredie, J.A., in,
    Proceedings of the Tenth International Cancer Congress,
    Houston, 1970.

91. Pisciotta, A.V., Westring, D.W., DePrey, C. and Walsh, B.
    Nature, *215*: 193, 1967.

92. Silk, M., Cancer, *20*: 2088, 1967.

93. Trubowittz, S., Maske, B., and Del Rosario, A., Cancer, *19*: 2019, 1966.

94. Al-Sarraf, M., Sardesai, S. and Vaitekevicius, V., Cancer, *27*: 1426, 1971.

95. Edwards, A.J., Rowland, G.F. and Lee, M.R., Lancet, *1*: 687, 1973.

96. Sucio-Foca, N., Buda, J.A., LoGerfo, P., Moulton, A., Weber, C., Wheeler, B. and Reemtsma, K., Oncology, *29*: 219, 1974.

97. Glasgow, A.H., Nimberg, R.D., Menzoian, J.O., Saporoschetz, I., Cooperband, S.R., Schmid, K., Mannick, J.A., New Eng. J. Med., *291;* 1263, 1974.

98. Glasgow, A.H., Menzoian, J.O., Nimberg, R.D., Cooperband, S.R., Schmid, K., and Mannick, J.A., Surgery, *76*: 35, 1974.

99. Veit, B.C. and Michael, J.G., Nature New Biol., *235*: 238, 1972.

100. Lindahl,-Magnusson, P., Leary, P. and Gresser, I., Nature New Biol., *237*: 120, 1972.

101. Rozee, K.R., Lee, S.H.S. and Ngan, J., Nature New Biol., *245*: 16, 1973.

102. Hirsch, M.D., Ellis, D.A., Black, P.H., Monaco, A.P. and Wood, M.L., Transplantation, *17*: 234, 1974.

103. Hirsch, M.S., Ellis, D.A., Proffitt, M.P., Black, P.H. and Chirigos, M.A., Nature New Biol., *244*: 102, 1973.

104. Chester, T.J., Paucker, K. and Merigan, T.C., Nature New Biol., *246*: 92, 1973.

105. Thorbecke, G.J., Friedman-Kein, A.E. and Vilcek, J., Cellular Immunol., *12*: 290, 1974.

106. Bullock, W.W. and Möller, E., Europ. J. Immunol., *2*: 514, 1972.

107. Benson, M.D., Aldo-Benson, M.A., Shirahama, T.,
     Borel, Y. and Cohen, A.S., J. Exp. Med., *142*: in
     press, 1975.

108. Nelson, D.S. and Schneider, C.W., Europ. J. Immunol.,
     4: 79, 1974.

109. Burger, D.R., Lilley, D.P. and Vetto, R.M., Cellular
     Immunol., *19*: 432, 1974.

110. Takada, A., Yumiko, T. and Minowada, J., J. Exp. Med.,
     140: 538, 1974.

111. Watson, J., J. Immunol., *111*: 1301, 1973.

112. Vann, D.C. and Galloway, P.C., J. Immunol., *110*: 1542,
     1973.

113. Vann, D.C. and Dotson, C.R., J. Immunol., *112*: 1149,
     1974.

114. Armerding, D. and Katz, D.H., J. Exp. Med., *140*: 19,
     1974.

115. Armerding, D., Sachs, D.H. and Katz, D.H., J. Exp. Med.,
     140: 1717, 1974.

116. Rich, R.R. and Pierce, C.W., J. Immunol., *112*: 1360,
     1974.

117. Danielson, J.R. and Val Alten, P.J., Progr. Exp. Tumor
     Research, *19*: 194, 1974.

118. Green, S.S. and Sell, K.W., *In Vitro*, *8*: 396, 1973.

119. Green, S.S., Wistar, R. Jr., and Sell, K.W.,
     Transplantation, *18*: 496, 1974.

120. Anderson, J., Sjöberg, O., and Möller, G., Transplant.
     Rev., *11*: 131, 1972.

121. Gorczynski, R.M., Miller, R.G. and Phillips, R.A.,
     J. Immunol., *110*: 968, 1973.

122. Doria, G., Agarossi, G. and DiPietro, S., J. Immunol.,
     108: 268, 1972.

123. Waldman, H. and Munro, A., Nature, *253*: 356, 1973.

124. Kishimoto, T. and Ishizaka, K., J. Immunol., *112*: 1685, 1974.

125. Waldman, S.R. and Gottlieb, A.A., Cellular Immunol., *9*: 142, 1973.

126. Nelson, D.S., Nature, *246*: 306, 1973.

127. Calderon, J., Williams, R.T. and Unanue, E.R., Proc. Nat. Acad. Sci., *71*: 4273, 1974.

128. Opitz, H.G., Niethammer, D., Lemke, H., Flad, H.D. and Huget, R., Cellular Immunol., *16*: 379, 1975.

129. Perkins, E.H. and Makinodan, T., J. Immunol., *94*: 765, 1965.

130. Parkhouse, R.M.E., and Dutton, R.W., J. Immunol., *97*: 663, 1966.

131. Moore, R.D. and Schoenberg, M.D., Nature, *219*: 297, 1968.

132. Diener, E., Shortman, K. and Russel, P., Nature, *225*: 731, 1970.

133. Cone, L. and Uhr, J.W., J. Clin. Invest., *43*: 2241, 1964.

134. Zolla, S., J. Immunol., *108*: 1039, 1972.

135. Tanapatchaiyapong, P. and Zolla, S., Science, *186*: 748, 1974.

136. Riggio, R.R., Parrillo, J.E. Jr., Bull, F.G., Schwartz, G.H., Stenzel, K.H. and Rubin, A.L., Transplantation, *12*: 400, 1971.

137. Ogra, S.S., Murgita, R.A. and Tomasi, T.B. Jr., Immunol Communications, *3*: 497, 1974.

138. Schumaker, K., Maerker-Alzer, G. and Wehmer, U., Nature, *251*: 655, 1974.

139. Sample. W.F., Gertner, H.R. Jr., and Chretien, P.B., J. Nat. Cancer Inst., *46*: 1291, 1971.

140. Gatti, R.A., Lancet, *1*: 1351, 1971.

141. Steward, A.M., J. Nat. Cancer Inst., *50*: 625, 1973.

142. Apffel, G.A., Arneson, B.G., Twiman, C.W. and Harris, C.A., Brit. J. Cancer, *20*: 122, 1966.

143. McCarthy, R.E., Coffin, J.N. and Gates, S.L., Transplantation, *6*: 737, 1968.

144. Kamo, I. and Ishida, N., Gann, *62*: 453, 1971.

145. Chan, P.L., Sinclair, N.R. St. C., J. Nat. Cancer Inst., *48*: 1629, 1972.

146. Moscarelli, P., Villi, M.L., Garotta, G., Porta, C., Bigi, G. and Clerici, E., J. Immunol., *111*: 977, 1973.

147. Frost, P. and Lance, E.M., Nature, *246*: 101, 1973.

148. Hrsak, I. and Marotti, T., Europ. J. Cancer. *9*: 717, 1973.

149. Yamazaki, H., Nitta, K. and Umezawa, H., Gann, *64*: 83, 1973.

150. Motoki, H., Kamo, I., Kikuchi, M., Ono, Y. and Ishida, N., Gann, *65*: 269, 1974.

151. Anderson, R.J., McBride, C.M. and Hersh, E.M., Cancer Research, *32*: 988, 1972.

152. Gillette, R.W. and Boone, C.W., J. Nat. Cancer Inst., *50*: 1391, 1973.

153. Wong, A., Mankovita, R. and Kennedy, J.C., Europ. J. Cancer Inst., *13*: 530, 1974.

154. Bonmasser, E., Bonmasser, A., Goldin, A. and Cudkowicz, G., Cancer Research, *33*: 1054, 1973.

155. Kamo, I., Patel, C., Kateley, J., and Friedman, H., J. Nat. Cancer Inst., in press, 1975.

DISCUSSION FOLLOWING PRESENTATION

by DR. SIDNEY R. COOPERBAND

G. SISKIND: What is the normal concentration of the alpha
globulin inhibitor in the serum?

S. COOPERBAND: I wish I could answer you. I honestly cannot
tell you. We know that in a preparation of the
fraction IV material we have concentrated it 200 to 500
fold. However, we also know that our ability to isolate
the material varies. We lose it on filters and on
surfaces. I really do not know the normal concentration
of the material.

G. SISKIND: Would you think the normal concentration is in
the microgram range or the milligram range?

S. COOPERBAND: I would think the microgram range. Other
people have isolated materials (extracts of tissues)
which appear to function in the same way as ours, but
are active at 1-2 µg/ml. By "appear to function in the
same way" I mean that these inhibitors are only active
when added before antigen. We have never had preparations which were active at such levels. Our best
preparations are active at 50 µg/ml.

C. LAINE: When you isolate the suppressive activity is there
any suppressive activity left behind, or do you see the
unmasking of some stimulating activity?

S. COOPERBAND: We have not as yet completely removed suppressive activity from any material. We find some sera
which do not have detectable suppressive antibody but
from which we can isolate suppressive activity after
fractionation. We then find that if you isolate the
suppressive peptide from it you do not remove all

suppressive activity. We have occassionally found something left behind which is stimulatory but this finding
is very inconsistent.

C. LAINE: Do you have any idea about the mechanism of action?

S. COOPERBAND: Based on the fact that it is absorbed very
    poorly and can be washed off very easily, we suggest
    that it must act on the cell surface. The fact that
    you can reverse its effect fairly soon after removal
    also suggests that it is a cell surface event. We have
    examined the effect of the suppressive material on
    antigen binding. I did not show any of this data
    because I am not satisfied with it. The data are
    rather strange. We inhibit antigen binding by about
    50%. I do not understand that. I am not satisfied that
    the experiments were done properly. We studied antigen
    binding by two methods: (a) using antigen-coated-
    tanned-erythrocytes, and (b) using antigen binding at
    equilibrium. In both of these systems suppressive doses
    of alpha globulin depress antigen binding by about 50%.
    I do not really understand these results.

GUPTA: Can you block the suppressive effect by any procedure?

S. COOPERBAND: We have so far been unable to reverse it with
    a number of agents.

GUPTA: Is there a receptor for the suppressor globulin on
    the T cells, perhaps close to the activation site?

S. COOPERBAND: We did some pharmacologic experiments which
    are analagous to competative antagonism type studies.
    Pharmacologically there appeared to be a type of
    antagonism suggesting two separate receptors on the
    surface of the cell for either antigen or mitogen and
    for the alpha globulin. The second receptor does not
    appear to compete directly or noncompetitively. It
    appears to be a pharmacologic competition. It appears
    to be a distant site which interferes with binding.

O'REILLY: Is the suppressor alpha globulin a fat carrying
    protein? There have been reports that serum from hyper-
    lipemic patients can suppress the response to PHA.

S. COOPERBAND: No! Fraction IV contains a high concentra-
    tion of alpha-1-lipoprotein. We early found it
    necessary to delipidize it in order to simplify handling
    of the material. We extracted it with ether and removed
    the lipid without loss of activity.

QUESTION: Since the peptide was found in immunized
    mice, could you find it in immunized humans?

S. COOPERBAND: First it was not the peptide isolated by
    Viet Michael. They found an alpha globulin protein.
    They did not isolate a peptide. Their protein is
    somewhat different from the material we are studying.
    Their material is thermally unstable at 56-60°C while
    our material is stable up to 80°C. We are looking at
    the serum, not so much in immunized humans, as in
    patients who are undergoing a series of inflammatory
    insults. The data are not all in as yet but they
    suggest that the material is present in anyone who has
    an inflammatory insult.

GOLDMAN: Can the activity be destroyed by any enzymes?
    Does it have species specificity?

S. COOPERBAND: It is inhibited by chymotrypsin and pronase
    but not by trypsin.

    Field and Caspary have reported the isolation of an
    $alpha_2$-macroglobulin from patients with cancer. They
    were able to dissociate from that globulin, by
    disulfide rupture, a peptide with suppressive activity.
    We have seen batches of $alpha_2$- macroglobulin which are
    suppressive and others which are not suppressive. Thus,
    we don't find any correlation between $alpha_2$-macro-
    globulin and suppression.

    The material appears to have similar activity when
    tested in different species. We routinely test the

human material in the mouse, and mouse suppressive
material in the guinea pig and they are all suppressive
to roughly the same extent. There may be a slight dose
dependency in favor of the species of origin. That is,
they may be slightly more effective in the species of
origin.

RAND: Does the suppressor material have any effect on intra-
cellular cyclic-AMP or GMP or on adenyl cyclase
activity?

S. COOPERBAND: We are now studying this. We have done
three experiments and find roughly a doubling of adenyl
cyclase activity in lymphocytes within five minutes
after exposure.

R. SHANDAR: What type of testing did you do before calling
cancer patients anergic?

S. COOPERBAND: They were tested with a battery of recall
antigens plus DNCB.

STONER: Does the suppressive material effect capping?

S. COOPERBAND: We have not looked at the effect of alpha
globulin on capping. The only thing we have looked at
is its effect on the kinetics of binding and we find
that it reduces the total antigen bound. This occurs
even at $4^{\circ}C$.

SUNSHINE: Is it possible to demonstrate that low doses of
alpha gloublin are stimulatory and high doses are
suppressive?

S. COOPERBAND: The early batches often gave considerable
stimulation at low concentrations but it was not a
completely consistent finding. We haven't looked at
this possible effect with the polypeptide.

SUNSHINE: Do you see accelerated graft rejection at low
    doses?

S. COOPERBAND: We have not looked.

B- and T-CELL FUNCTION IN MALIGNANT LYMPHOMA

Alan C. Aisenberg

*John Collins Warren Laboratories
of the Huntington Memorial Hospital
of Harvard University at The Massachusetts General Hospital
Boston, Massachusetts*

INTRODUCTION

Rapid progress in understanding the disease mechanisms which underlie the lymphomas and lymphocytic leukemias was to be expected since these neoplasms result from aberrant growth and function of the lymphocyte, the cell which has dominated modern immunology. Central to an exposition of immunity in lymphoid malignancy is the division of lymphocytes into B and T cells {reviewed in Davies and Carter (1)} which has followed directly from the elucidation of thymus function. Table I summarizes some of the recent information about B and T lymphocytes.

Both B and T cells arise in the bone marrow and both are morphologically small lymphocytes. The B cell reaches the lymphoid organs without passage through the thymus, and is an effector cell which produces antibody and is concerned primarily with humoral immunity. Its localization is characteristically in the follicles of the lymph nodes and spleen, and it comprises a minority of the small lymphocytes in the blood, lymph and lymphoid organs. The T lymphocyte finds its way to the lymph nodes and spleen only after transit through and processing by the thymus. This cell constitutes the majority population of small lymphocytes of blood and lymphoid organs, and is principally located in the interfollicular cortex of the lymph nodes and the periarterial sheath of the spleen. The T cell is an intermediate or helper cell interposed between antigen and the effector B lymphocyte. The T cell is concerned particularly with the

TABLE I

Properties of B and T Lymphocytes

Property	B Lymphocytes	T Lymphocytes
Origin	bone marrow	bone marrow
Destination	lymph nodes and spleen	lymph nodes and spleen
Intermediate stop	direct ?	thymus
Circulates via	blood (20-30% of lymphocytes) lymph, thoracic duct	blood (70-80% of lymphocytes) lymph, thoracic duct
Morphology	small lymphocyte	small lymphocyte
Function	effector cell antibody-forming cell antibody formation (IgM>IgG)	intermediate or helper cell; antigen-reactive cell; cellular immunity (graft-*vs*-host reaction, bacterial allergy, contact sensitivity, homograft reaction, antitumor immunity); secondary role in antibody formation (IgG>IgM), particularly response to particulate antigens such as sheep erythrocytes.

	plasma cell	immunoblast
Differentiates into	plasma cell	immunoblast
Localization		
Lymph nodes	primary and secondary follicles medullary cords	interfollicular cortex (paracortex)
Spleen	primary and secondary follicles marginal zone	periarterial sheath
Properties		
Surface Ig	+	−
Thymus-specific antigens	−	+
Receptors for Ig and complement	+	−
Rosette formation with sheep RBC	−	+
Response to PHA	−	+
Retention by nylon	+	−

various cell-mediated immune reactions (graft-*versus*-host
and homograft reactions, bacterial and contact sensitivity,
delayed hypersensitivity and many forms of antitumor
immunity), though it is also implicated in the antibody
response to certain antigens.

B and T lymphocytes can be distinguished by a number of
cell surface characteristics. An important characteristic
of the B cell is the presence of large amounts of immunoglobulin on the cell surface which can be demonstrated by
the fluorescent antibody technique: T cells lack detectable
surface immunoglobulin. B lymphocytes also have receptors
for complement and for immunoglobulin and a high affinity for
nylon fiber columns, while T cells possess thymus-specific
markers on their surface, respond to phytohemagglutinin and
form rosettes with sheep erythrocytes.

IMMUNOLOGICAL REACTIONS IN HODGKIN'S DISEASE

Historical Background.

The largest part of this article is devoted to the
immunological reactions in Hodgkin's disease since most of
the immunological investigations in lymphoma and leukemia
deal with this disorder. Indeed, the immune status of the
patients with Hodgkin's disease has generated a minor
polemic.

The early studies of Parker *et al.* and Steiner {see
Eisenberg for references (2)} unexpectedly disclosed a high
incidence of tuberculin negativity in patients with Hodgkin's
disease. However, it was only after Schier's observations in
the 1950's (3) that tuberculin negativity was recognized to be
a manifestation of impaired cellular immunity that Hodgkin's
disease patients were found unreactive to the entire spectrum
of intradermal skin test antigens of the bacterial or delayed
type (mumps skin test antigen, streptokinase/streptodornase,
tuberculin, Candida and Trichophyton). A reasonably correct
assessment of the immune deficiency was possible in the mid
1960's when active sensitization with dinitrochlorbenzene
(DNCB) was introduced to study these individuals. This is
because intradermal testing evaluates past sensitivities

rather than the ability to acquire new sensitivities. With appropriate testing these defects can now be placed in the perspective (Table II) of impaired thymus-mediated lymphocyte function (2,4).

Controversy arose when the authors of an otherwise exemplary study of immunity in patients with untreated Hodgkin's disease (5) chose increasingly to stress the fraction of patients reacting normally, rather than the experimental difficulty in establishing the presence of a minor degree of immune impairment. Several recent studies, equally meticulous in execution, indicate that, when sufficient care is exercised, minor impairment of skin sensitivity (6,7) and lymphocyte reactivity (8,9) can be recognized in most patients with untreated Hodgkin's disease of limited anatomical extent.

It is convenient to discuss the immune impairment of Hodgkin's disease under three categories: untreated patients, treated patients in good clinical condition, and patients in poor condition with far advanced disease. Dividing the subject in this way has the added benefit of stressing the progressive nature of the immune deficiency.

Untreated Patients.

A subtle defect in cellular immunity (6), easily over-looked, can be demonstrated by active sensitization with dinitrochlorobenzene in about 80 percent of patients with untreated Hodgkin's disease. However, the defect can only be demonstrated by attenuating the antigenic stimulus (the concentration of DNCB) to a level at which 15-20 percent of normal controls fail to react. The immune deficiency can also be observed when a reduced concentration of strepto-kinase/streptodornase is employed as an interdermal (recall) antigen. These DNCB studies were originally criticized because radiation therapy was begun in many individuals between the time of DNCB sensitization and subsequent testing for sensitivity two weeks later. It remains possible that laparotomy, which is frequently performed during the two-week hiatus, may influence the results.

TABLE II

Thymus Dependent Immunity and Hodgkin's Disease *

	Thymectomized Animal	Hodgkin's Disease Patient
A. Cellular Immunity		
1. Homograft reaction	↓	↓
2. Graft-*vs*-host reaction	↓	↓(lymphocyte transfer reaction)
3. Delayed hypersensitivity		
a) Bacterial	↓	↓
b) Contact	↓	↓
4. Lymphocytes		
a) Number	↓ to about 40% normal, loss of long-lived cells	↓
b) Transformation	↓	↓
B. Humoral Immunity		
1. Immunoglobulin levels	N	N or ↑, except late ↓(IgM>IgG)
2. Plasma cells	N	N
3. Antibody formation	N to ↓	N to ↓
	a) BSA>ShC>Pneumo.,Fer.,Hemo.	a) Typhoid, Tet.>Pneumo.
	b) Primary>Secondary	b) Primary>Secondary
	c) IgG>IgM	

C. Infection

Wasting in newborn.
Protection by germ-free
environment.
Susceptibility to hepatitis
virus.

Susceptibility to various viral,
fungal, protozoal and bacterial
agents, often of low patho-
genicity; Herpes group (CMV, H.
Zoster), Torula, Histoplasma,
Candida, Nocardia, Pneumocystis,
Listeria, etc., etc.

* *N = normal; ↓ = decreased or impaired; > = more impaired than; BSA = bovine serum
albumin; ShC = sheep erythrocytes; Pneumo. = pneumococcus polysaccharide;
Fer. = ferritin; Hemo. = hemocyanin; Tet. = tetanus toxoid; CMV = cytomegalovirus.*

There is ample residual cellular immunity in such
untreated Hodgkin's disease patients, and infections related
to the deficiency are rarely seen at this time. The presence
of immune impairment at the onset of the disorder does not
appear to be of prognostic value, at least for the five or
so years of available follow-up (5), and the fraction of
unreactive patients appears to be independent of the extent
of disease (6).

Absolute lymphocyte counts in untreated patients (6)
tend to be at the lower end of the normal range or slightly
below the lower limit (levels of 1000-2000 per mm^3 are
usually observed in untreated Hodgkin's disease compared with
a normal range of 1500-3000 per mm^3). Although there is some
argument, lymphopenia is probably more severe in the presence
of advanced disease and the so-called lymphocyte depletion
histopathologic subtype. By meticulous control of the phytohemagglutinin concentration (9) or by following the entire
time course of the *in vitro* reaction (8), peripheral blood
lymphocytes from most patients with untreated Hodgkin's
disease can be shown to be less reactive than cells from
normal controls. However, depression of this T-cell function
is quite subtle, with considerable overlap between normal
and disease populations. The degree of impaired phytohemagglutinin responsiveness appears to be related to the extent
of the disorder, but unresponsiveness persists for several
years, at least, after successful treatment of Hodgkin's
disease (9). There have been reports of decreased T lymphocytes in the blood as measured by rosette formation, but
there appears to be no gross depletion of T cells from the
peripheral blood of untreated patients. It is more likely
that the impairment of cellular immunity of these early
patients results from either a loss of a T-cell subpopulation
or a functional impairment of the T lymphocyte.

Normal lymphocyte reactivity has been observed in some
patients with depressed skin reactions, raising the
possibility that the immune deficit may not result solely
from defective lymphocyte function (10); there is evidence
that the inflammatory response may be reduced in some
patients with Hodgkin's disease. It has also been found that
lymphocytes from patients with this disorder exhibit an
enhanced level of blast transformation and associated DNA
synthesis prior to the addition of a stimulant such as phytohemagglutinin (11). The significance of this observation is

obscure, but it has been taken as evidence of some form of
ongoing immune reaction, perhaps to the etiologic agent
responsible for the disorder.

Treated Patients in Good Clinical Condition.

Most individuals in good clinical condition who are
under medical observation because of active Hodgkin's disease
have a defect in cellular immunity easily demonstrated by
their inability to acquire sensitivity to DNCB (4) and their
unreactivity to a variety of delayed-type intradermal skin
test antigens (3,12,13). The humoral response to many
antigens appears normal, but it is likely that a minor
defect in antibody formation is present (4,14) on the basis
of the observed loss of the primary response to some antigens
(a deficiency similar to that seen in thymectomized animals)
and diminution in the duration of the primary response to
others. Lymphocyte counts tend to be lower in treated
patients than in untreated, and depression of the reactivity
of lymphocytes *in vitro* is more easily demonstrated (15).
Rejection of skin homografts may be impaired, and the
reaction of lymphocytes transferred from patients to the skin
of other individuals (the lymphocyte transfer reaction) is
depressed. In the treated patient, in contrast to those who
have not received treatment, the presence of obvious immune
impairment appears to be of prognostic significance; i.e.,
patients with active Hodgkin's disease whose negative tuberculin status cannot be converted by B.C.G. vaccination have
a markedly poorer outlook than those who can be converted
(16).

There is little question that radiation therapy and the
various cytotoxic drugs employed in the treatment of
Hodgkin's disease can cause an immunological deficit similar
to that seen in the disorder itself (17). However, the
persistent residue of immune impairment from radiation and
intermittant drug treatment is modest, and it seems likely
that the disease rather than its treatment is the more
important factor in most patients with active disease. For
example, immunologically impaired individuals who respond
favorably to MOPP (nitrogen mustard, Oncovin, procarbazine
and prednisone) combination chemotherapy, rapidly regain
their cellular immune responses. Similarly, it is unlikely
that either vinblastine or procarbazine as currently employed

are potent immunosuppressants. For the most part, patients with active disease in good clinical state who are not taking adrenal corticoids are usually not at great risk for the development of opportunistic infections.

Patients in Poor Condition with Advanced Hodgkin's Disease.

All patients in whom the disease process cannot be irradicated by treatment eventually experience deterioration of general health because of progressive and spreading lymphoma. Profound impairment of all parameters of cellular immune function is obvious in such individuals. Antibody formation may be deficient and serum immunoglobulin levels, particularly the level of IgM, may fall (18). Lymphopenia may be extreme with almost complete absence of small lymphocytes from the peripheral blood smear. Continuous treatment particularly with the adrenal corticosteroids, but probably with other cytotoxic drugs as well, contributes to the severe and often fatal infections observed in such patients with end stage Hodgkin's disease {Table II, (19)}. Viruses, fungi, and bacteria of low virulence which require intact cell mediated defense mechanisms are the characteristic infectious agents, though the more usual bacterial pathogens are also frequently seen.

Significance of the Immunological Defect.

Allowing that a derangement of T-cell mediated immunity is a frequent finding in patients with untreated Hodgkin's disease of limited anatomical extent, the significance of the defect in the pathogenesis of the disorder requires comment. Perhaps the most plausible explanation for the deficiency postulates that the T lymphocyte is the site at which the etiologic agent of Hodgkin's disease acts; by direct observation most of the lymphocytes of the Hodgkin's disease lymph node are T lymphocytes. The hypothetical agent might subvert T-cell function throughout the body, but produce anatomical evidence of Hodgkin's disease in only one or a few sites. Such a view is consonant with a viral etiology of the disorder, a view which continues to enjoy widespread acceptance despite the elusiveness of direct proof. Indirect support for the hypothesis comes from the observation that many viral infections, including measles and even measles

vaccination with attenuated virus, produce cellular immune
impairment similar to that seen in Hodgkin's disease. However, the immune defect observed in Hodgkin's disease can
hardly serve as definitive proof of the site at which the
etiologic agent acts, and certainly not as evidence of a
viral etiology. There is little at present to recommend the
view that T-cell impairment is the primary event and that the
diagnostic morphological changes of the disorder are
secondary phenomena.

IMMUNOLOGICAL REACTION IN OTHER LYMPHOMAS
AND LYMPHOCYTIC LEUKEMIAS

Host immunity in lymphoid neoplasms other than Hodgkin's
disease has not been studied systematically. Testing of
cellular immunity and antibody production has been done, for
the most part, without sufficient regard to the lymphoma
subtype and prior treatment. Only a few studies of the past
decade (20-22) have been sufficiently stringent in these
regards. However, an important new line of investigation has
developed from the study of the cell surface of neoplastic
lymphocytes. Analysis of these cells for the surface
properties listed at the bottom of Table I has permitted the
determination of the B or T-cell lineage of the neoplastic
cells in many lymphoproliferative disorders (23,24).

*Chronic Lymphocytic Leukemia (CLL) and Well Differentiated
Lymphocytic Lymphoma (Lymphocytic Lymphoma).*

Except for Hodgkin's disease, the lymphoproliferative
disorder which has received most careful immunologic
scrutiny is chronic lymphocytic leukemia. It is usually
assumed that well differentiated lymphocytic lymphoma
represents a nonleukemic variant of the same pathological
process as that of CLL, and many studies do not separate the
findings obtained in the two disorders.

A considerable amount of recent experimental evidence
indicates that CLL is a proliferation of B lymphocytes. In
common with normal B lymphocytes, cells from about 90 percent
of CLL patients have immunoglobulin on the cell surface which

can be readily demonstrated with the fluorescent antibody
technique (23,24). Unlike normal B cells, analysis of the
surface immunoglobulin shows the cells to be clonal, i.e.,
the Ig on all cells from a single patient is of a single
heavy chain type and a single light chain type. CLL cells
have many other B cell properties {see Aisenberg (25) for
references}; unresponsiveness to phytohemagglutinin,
inability to form rosettes with sheep erythrocytes, the
presence of receptors for complement and immunoglobulin,
retention by nylon fibers, absence of thymus-specific markers
and a complex villous pattern on scanning electron micros-
copy.

The immune defect of CLL contrasts with that of
Hodgkin's disease, i.e., B-lymphocyte-mediated humoral
immunity is lost early in CLL. Thus, immunoglobulin levels
decline, the antibody response to test antigens is impaired,
and there is marked susceptibility to pyogenic bacterial
pathogens such as the pneumococcus, i.e., organisms in which
protection is mediated via humoral rather than cellular
immune mechanisms. Cellular immunity appears to be pre-
served at the onset of CLL as evidenced by intact skin
reactions to the usual recall antigens (tuberculin, etc.),
though the evidence is divided about whether the ability to
acquire new skin sensitivities (to dinitrofluorobenzene) is
completely normal (20,21). Presumably, the neoplastic B
lymphocyte replaces the normal B-cell population, thus sub-
verting B-cell function. Later in the course of CLL and
allied disorders, drug treatment frequently superimposes a
T-cell deficit.

*Poorly Differentiated Lymphocytic Lymphoma (Lymphoblastic
Lymphoma).*

Application of cell surface study to this disorder
indicates that it too is a B-cell proliferation, but the
cells differ from the small mature lymphocytes of CLL.
These "poorly differentiated" lymphocytes are usually
larger cells, frequently with cleaved nuclei, and display
much larger quantities of immunoglobulin on their surface
than is present on the CLL cell (23). It is probably that
the cells of most patients with lymphosarcoma cell leukemia
and nodular lymphoma belong to the same B-cell subtype as
the cell of poorly differentiated lymphocytic lymphoma.

Evidence is accumulating that this entire group of proliferations arises from special cells of the germinal center
termed germinocytes and germinoblasts (26). A second disorder of similar morphology is a T-cell proliferation which
arises in the thymus of children.

The medical literature gives little clear indication of
the state of host immunity in patients with these disorders.
It seems probably that individuals with early disease have
neither a prominent defect in cellular (T cell) or humoral
(B cell) immunity (12,13), but such a conclusion must be
tentative. As these disorders progress, treatment and
debility impose their toll on immune reactivity.

Other Lymphomas and Lymphoid Leukemias.

There is little definite data about the cell lineage or
immune status of histiocytic lymphoma (reticulum cell
sarcoma); indeed, it is not proven that this is in fact a
disorder of histiocytes. Preliminary evidence suggests that
acute lymphocytic leukemia is a T-cell proliferation, but the
infectious complications seen are caused by granulocyte
depletion and treatment rather than impairment of either B or
T cell immunity. Immunologically, acute lymphocytic leukemia
is not particularly lymphocytic, i.e., it resembles acute
granulocytic leukemia. Among rarities, the Sézary cell of
mycosis fungoides has been demonstrated to be a T lymphocyte,
but host immunity in this disorder appears to be intact.

SUMMARY

In the preceding discussion a simple pattern appears to
emerge. In Hodgkin's disease the early and characteristic
loss of T-cell mediated cellular immunity may reflect the
site at which the etiological agent is acting. Chronic lymphocytic leukemia and the closely allied well differentiated
lymphocytic lymphoma are B-cell proliferations in which B-
cell mediated humoral immunity is first depressed. Poorly
differentiated lymphocytic lymphoma is also a B-cell

proliferation, but the immune deficit, if present, has not been characterized. Acute lymphocytic leukemia (and probably the thymic lymphoma of children) may be of T-cell lineage, but granulocyte depletion and immunosuppressive antitumor therapy are the main causes of the immune defect seen. The immune reactions of histiocytic lymphoma remain to be clarified. Some of the foregoing statements are based on preliminary experimental data; the many new techniques now available should permit a rapid expansion of existing knowledge.

ACKNOWLEDGEMENTS

This is publication No. 1472 of the Cancer Commission of Harvard University.

REFERENCES

1. Davies, A.J.S. and Carter, R.L., Contemporary Topics in Immunol., *1*: 1, 1972.

2. Aisenberg, A.C., Cancer Res., *26*: 1152, 1966.

3. Schier, W.W., New Eng. J. Med., *250*: 353, 1954.

4. Aisenberg, A.C., J. Clin. Invest., *41*: 1964, 1962.

5. Young, R.C., Corder, M.P., Haynes, H.A. and DeVita, V.T. Am. J. Med., *52*: 63, 1972.

6. Eltringham, J.R. and Kaplan, H.S., U.S. Nat. Cancer Inst. Monograph, *36*: 107, 1973.

7. Gaines, J.D., Giliner, M.A. and Remington, J.S., U.S. Nat. Cancer Inst. Monograph, *36*: 117, 1973.

8. Matchett, K.M., Huang, A.T. and Kremer, W.B., J. Clin. Invest., *52*: 1908, 1973.

9. Levy, R. and Kaplan, H.S., New Eng. J. Med., *290*: 181, 1974.

10. Churchill, W.H., Rocklin, R.B., Moloney, W.C. and David, J.R., U.S. Nat. Cancer Inst. Monograph, *36*: 99, 1973.

11. Fairley, G.H., Crowther, D., Powles, R.L., Sewell, R.L. and Balchin, L.A., U.S. Nat. Cancer Inst. Monograph, *36*: 95, 1973.

12. Sokal, J.E. and Aungst, C.W., Cancer, *14*: 597, 1961.

13. Lamb, D., Pilney, F., Kelley, W.D. and Good, R.A., J. Immunol., *89*: 555, 1962.

14. Chase, M.W., Cancer Res., *26*: 1097, 1966.

15. Hersh, E.M. and Oppenhein, J.J., New Eng. J. Med., *273*: 1006, 1965.

16. Sokal, J.E. and Aungst, C.W., Cancer, *24*: 128, 1969.

17. Aisenberg, A.C., Adv. in Pharm. and Chemother., *8*: 31, 1970.

18. Goldman, J.M. and Hobbs, J.R., Immunology, *13*: 421, 1967

19. Casazza, A.R., Davall, C.P. and Carbone, P.P., Cancer Res., *26*: 1290, 1966.

20. Cone, L. and Uhr, J.W., J. Clin. Invest., *43*: 2241, 1964

21. Block, J.B., Haynes, H.A., Thompson, W.L. and Herman, P.E., J. Nat. Cancer Inst., *42*: 973, 1969.

22. Miller, D.G., in *Immunological Diseases* (Second Edition) Edited by M. Samter, D.W. Talmage, B. Rose, W.B. Sherman and J.H. Vaughan, p. 548, Little, Brown and Co., Boston, 1971.

23. Aisenberg, A.C., Bloch, K.J. and Long, J.C., Am. J. Med. *55*: 184, 1973.

24. Seligmann, M., Preudhomme, J.-L. and Brouet, J.-C.,
    Transplant. Rev., *16*: 85, 1973.

25. Aisenberg, A.C., Human Path., *4*: 301, 1973.

26. Lukes, R.J. and Collins, R.D., Gann Monograph on Cancer
    Res., *15*: 209, 1973.

DISCUSSION FOLLOWING PRESENTATION

by DR. ALAN C. AISENBERG

N. MACRIS: Were you using a specific antiserum or a poly-
     valent antiserum for identification of B cells by
     fluorescence microscopy?

A. AISENBERG: Usually we work with specific antisera. It
     was not just a polyvalent antiserum. There is no
     question that the CLL cells can be either IgM or IgG
     bearing. The IgM CLL's are much more frequent, on the
     order of 6:1. The IgG bearing cells lack IgM. They are
     clonal in that they bear either a κ or λ light chain.
     The "brilliant" cells all appear to be IgM bearing. I
     have never seen any IgG bearing "brilliant" cells. They
     are also clonal in that they are either κ or λ in light
     chain type.

G. SISKIND: Do you find IgD bearing cells?

A. AISENBERG: In the first group we studied, we recorded
     that a few of our CLL's had a high percentage of IgD
     bearing cells. We did not have the necessary reagents
     at that time to be certain of the specificity. Since
     then there are a number of reports that IgD is
     frequently found with IgM. We have seen a couple of
     patients with leukemia who have IgD and no IgM. I have
     not seen enough of this latter type of patient to be
     certain. Small amounts of IgD is often present on cells
     with large amounts of IgM. The clonal nature (κ or λ
     light chains) is still maintained.

R. SHANDAR: With regard to the "brilliant" cells in CLL, is
     this related to temperature? At what temperature do you
     do your staining? Are the "brilliant" cells found in a
     different disease state?

A. AISENBERG: In CLL there is a problem in the definition
of the disease by the hematologist. I believe that if
you look at the lymph nodes in patients with "brilliant"
cells, they would look like lymph nodes of the various
types of non-Hodgkins lymphomas. The cell surface is
giving you a better assay of the species that is pro-
liferating in the particular disease than can be
obtained by the hematologist with the standard light
microscope. In summary, I believe that the three cases
with "brilliant" cells do not share certain charactis-
tics with the lymph nodes of the other 37 patients.
This is, however, only a prediction.

R. SHANDAR: What did you find in studying T-cell function in
the immunoglobulin negative CLL patients.

A. AISENBERG: There were four CLL patients who were immunoglobulin negative. These cells had complement
receptors, they did not react with antithymocyte
globulin, and they did not form sheep red blood cell
rosettes. Thus, I have never seen a true T-cell CLL
patient but as there are at least three such patients
reported they must occassionally occur.

What I am sure is happening is that the clinician
makes some very crude judgements about the nature of the
disease from what he sees under the light microscope and
that there are actually several different disease
states which he calls by the same name. Eventually,
this will sort out and probably one will see clinical
differences in these different groups of patients.

R. SHANDAR: Do you mean that those patients you described
that do not have surface immunoglobulins are actually
not CLL patients?

A. AISENBERG: What is CLL? It is a question of
definition. I think that those cases will show a
nodular lymphoma under the microscope. I further
believe that these patients have a different proliferation from that of the usual group of patients. This at
least is my guess.

G. SISKIND: That is, it appears as if you are now
      identifying different groups of patients in which
      different subpopulations of cells are involved. These
      patients probably should be regarded as having
      different disease states.